Normal

Normal

A Chaplain,
a Community with HIV/AIDS,
and the Eternal Life of Stories

AUDREY ELISA KERR

CASCADE *Books* • Eugene, Oregon

NORMAL
A Chaplain, a Community with HIV/AIDS, and the Eternal Life of Stories

Cascade Books
An Imprint of Wipf and Stock Publishers
199 W. 8th Ave., Suite 3
Eugene, OR 97401

www.wipfandstock.com

PAPERBACK ISBN: 978-1-5326-1340-1
HARDCOVER ISBN: 978-1-5326-1342-5
EBOOK ISBN: 978-1-5326-1341-8

Cataloguing-in-Publication data:

Names: Kerr, Audrey Elisa.

Title: Normal : A chaplain, a community with HIV/AIDS, and the eternal life of stories / Audrey Elisa Kerr.

Description: Eugene, OR: Cascade Books, 2018 | Includes bibliographical references.

Identifiers: ISBN 978-1-5326-1340-1 (paperback) | ISBN 978-1-5326-1342-5 (hardcover) | ISBN 978-1-5326-1341-8 (ebook)

Subjects: LCSH: AIDS (Disease)—Oral history. | Religion. | Health Policy. | Title.

Classification: RA644.A25 K455 2018 (print) | RA644 (ebook)

Manufactured in the U.S.A.   JUNE 13, 2018

Dedicated to:
Madison Alise and Maya Saybrook
and Gagi

Table of Contents

Acknowledgements

The program in Religion and the Arts at Yale Divinity School provided me with my first opportunity to explore narrative and spirituality as kindred disciplines. What an invaluable merger—this union of theology and creativity—and what a priceless gift it has been to me.

As a Coolidge Fellow with the Association for Religion in Intellectual Life I was able to receive valuable feedback from fellow scholars, pastors, and community advocates committed to merging social action, creativity, and religious life. I am thankful that I was a part of that vibrant and passionate cohort.

Being at home with the even and intelligent temperament of my then five-month-old baby allowed me to work on this manuscript. If anyone ever said that a baby is incompatible with writing, I would want them to meet baby Madison, even on her worst day. Moreover, Maya sat with me through various drafts, color coding my completed pages. Well done, Maya.

I would like to thank my family—Mary Kerr and the late Neville Kerr, my parents, and Jennifer Kerr Logan, my sister—for being there.

As always, I appreciate the presence of my closest comrades and confidants in the struggle to serve people with HIV and AIDS, especially the staff at the facility represented here. And, in the event that I never have another occasion to say it, I want to offer a long overdue thank you my teachers and mentors (past and present): Mr. Thomas Muratore, Rev. John T. Meehan, Dr. Barry Lee Pearson, Dr. Benjamin Barber, and the late Amiri Baraka. I'm also

ACKNOWLEDGEMENTS

grateful to the late poet Jayne Cortez who, along with Dr. Cheryl Wall, helped me get my first "real" job at PEN American Center.

My father was my first and most valuable reader, and it is difficult to write without his eyes traveling around my pages. I hope he is still journeying with me. Thank you, for everything.

And don't think the garden loses its ecstasy in winter.
It's quiet, but the roots are down there riotous.

—RUMI

Introduction

As I was writing this book, someone suggested to me that storytelling is the art form that most tethers us to this world. As listeners, it binds us to other humans. As storytellers, it frees us from the isolation that comes from withholding. And I was reminded at that moment that in the telling and the listening we do not just lift up voices: we center time, and define place, and better understand people; indeed, we immortalize our humanity, and the humanity of others.

As much as stories bind people together, each story is sovereign, retaining its own power and authority independent of the listeners. At the beginning of my journey as a chaplain, I had an inkling that stories would become my way of giving voice to a community whose identity was so often defined first and foremost by a debilitating disease. In all of the tragic, cerebral, comical, and incredulous ways I received them, I think I always knew that there were pieces of my patients' stories that I would share to secure eternal life for a community often steeped in the fragility of its mortality. I did not know at that time that autopathography—the way we tell stories in the midst of illness or disability—would ground my understanding of spiritual care.

That said, this book started even before that, and with a story that has long been forgotten by most. One hot summer morning, I was sitting in a rear pew at Riverside Cathedral on the Upper West Side of Manhattan. I was a research fellow in religion living in the enclaves of Columbia University. I'd long known Riverside to be home to bejeweled, elderly black women in blooming hats and animated, "churched" gay men. Everyone blended together there like nowhere else on Earth. On this morning, the morning of New York City's Gay Pride March, Rev. Dr. James Forbes, then pastor of Riverside, gave a sermon that reminded me of the power of the word to move mountains; it reminded me that it was the preacher as storyteller—not the politician, not the teacher—who was charged with imbuing the knowledge of social action into the spirit of a community.

Since this is a story about stories, I will share the first one first—courtesy of Rev. Forbes's sermon that Sunday.

Circa 1980, New York was at the beginning of the AIDS epidemic. The master narrative of the city was about individuals, then whole communities, progressing from a cough, to virulent diarrhea (then known as Gay Bowel Syndrome), to "gay-related cancers," to death—often in a matter of months, or weeks. These deaths were without historical precedent, without explanation or origin, agonizingly gruesome, intensely personal, and swift as bullets, targeting a historically marginalized community: gay men. Little was known about how one might catch the disease, or avoid it, or if it was entirely blood-borne, or saliva-borne, or communicable after death, and the terror that community members felt was palpable and urgent. It felt as if New York was battling the Bubonic plague of the twentieth century. And as the number of victims was rapidly outpacing the city's preparedness—or, more accurately, the limited willingness among New York service providers to assume the risk—the dead were often released to holding locations. The windows of vans carrying victims of AIDS-related deaths were blacked out, and families were often encouraged to accept cremation as the only option. Many funeral homes would not accept the ever-increasing numbers of bodies. Morgues that would take the bodies of AIDS victims were burdened beyond capacity. In that moment, without full knowledge of the risks or consequences, Riverside Church expanded itself spiritually, socially, and politically to include ministries, outreach, "calls to action," and sermons designed to create a home for the unwelcomed. Whether the disease was airborne, saliva-borne, or blood-borne, it was the work of the church to house souls and speak truth to power. Riverside, through funerals, ministries, activism, and support groups, became one of many spaces giving voice to the story of being HIV-positive in New York and, in this regard, it rescued bodies from both stigma and isolation. Of course they were far from alone in this effort, but what I wish to record here is that my desire to be an HIV/AIDS caregiver was not sparked by a medical interest, nor did it originate from personal kinship with people living with HIV/AIDS. My decision to serve was sparked by this story of radical hospitality.

For the last three decades of the twentieth century, HIV/AIDS was the health and human crisis that stood at the ground zero of marginalized people in a way that made it impossible for us to look away from health disparities, political disempowerment, economic inequality, social displacement, and sexuality, all dynamics I knew—as a professor of Black literature—to be also at the nexus of the marginalization of Black bodies in America. The purpose of this book is to use narratives to creative an ethnographic composite of a community of people with AIDS in a large, urban enclave, as I observed it as the chaplain of an HIV/AIDS care facility over the course of five years. I use the normative structures established through autopathography, a genre that focuses on the impact of terminal illness, chronic illness, or disability on the way an individual relates his or her story. The term *autopathograpy* was coined in 1997 by G. Thomas Couser in his seminal work *Recovering Bodies*. His work establishes the uniqueness of narratives rooted in illness and disability and creates a framework for future studies that address the body as a political landscape. Rather than imagining narratives as stories that advance stigmatization, Couser's understanding of narrative broadens the definition of "normal" by expanding our human connectedness to misunderstood bodies.[1]

As a professor, I want to co-opt social justice poetics—and as a chaplain, the living message of religious action—to suggest that listening to people who are ill is a process that itself disrupts the comfort of "othering" illness.

I am interested in the two unique "conditions" that impact the narratives of people living with HIV/ AIDS. The first condition is the disease itself, which—given that it is the most stigmatized illness of our generation—presents new opportunities to confront the social problem of the isolated self. The second condition is HIV/ AIDS narratives as a form of agency: for this disease, the very act of storytelling becomes a form of political and social intervention and empowerment. As one writer notes, AIDS presents "a sort of social x-ray of who is classified as mainstream and peripheral, deviant and normal," such that in the "scientific use and abuse of the 'promiscuities' paradigms, the accusations of responsibility for AIDS to homosexuals, is a case in point of this social x-ray."[2] Many AIDS patients claim membership in one or more of these "x-rayed groups." I would be remiss if I did not note that this disease moved fluidly through intersections of people who, even without AIDS, lived on the periphery of society, including the poor, women of color, the LGBTQ community, and drug abusers.

In some ways, HIV/ AIDS exacerbated boundaries between the center and the margins, but among those who are positive (some would argue), it "leveled cultural differences."[3] HIV/AIDS is the only illness of our time that is as social, political, and economic as it is medical. It is unique in its moral implications -- it is often transmitted through sexual intercourse or drug use -- and in its enigmatic nature, including its sudden appearance in the late 1970s and its growth into a pandemic. That said, one can look at any community that services people with AIDS in America—from a homeless shelter, to HIV/AIDS support groups, to treatment

1. Couser, *Recovering Bodies*, 8.
2. Herdt and Lindenbaum, *The Time of AIDS*, 8–9.
3. Ibid., 4.

clinics—and see that there are overlapping playing fields in the world of HIV/AIDS, but they are not equal. In this new millennium, this disease disproportionately ravages enclaves that are poor, drug addicted, or peopled by black and brown bodies.

This book is divided into five central sections, all of which attempt to allow stories told by and about this facility's residents to speak to the challenges that still surround living with HIV and AIDS. This book is hardly a *tour d' horizon* of living with HIV and AIDS; the scope is far more restrictive. It is intentionally limited to a particular place, during a limited time, and focusing on a few residents.

Moreover, I look at autopathography through the lens of my experience as chaplain and, in that regard, there are a few elements that distinguish this study from the plethora of contemporary HIV-related works across disciplinary orientations. First, I do not rigidly define this project as academic research, in that it does not seek to propose or answer a specific set of queries, adhere to prescribed methodological approaches, or offer a prescriptive agenda alongside a theoretically deduced evaluation. This project is a spiritual care memoir embedded in illness narratives that arose as I learned how to be a chaplain—how to hear stories and how to be heard, how to be both empathetic and spiritually helpful. This story required me to stand within the community's narratives as I unpeeled spiritual questions and confronted my shortcomings, and also as I sifted through the plethora of residents' needs, spiritual and otherwise.

Second, the facility represented here is a skilled nursing facility specifically for people with HIV/AIDS (one of a few such facilities in the country). Therefore, the presentation of the disease is not within the context of society-at-large, but in the context of *stages of this illness within a particular community*. The outcome, therefore, is a collection of narratives that explore the social, moral, and interpersonal patterns of everyday life while keeping an eye on the political, economic, gendered, and racial politics that are driving this disease beyond the facility. Indeed, this project sits at the intersection of the politics and the poetics of storytelling.

Third, while HIV is a chronic illness, the people I worked with were often closer to the end of their lives; in that regard, my experience is not reflective of the comparatively optimistic prospects for most people living with HIV/AIDS in America now.

The National Institute of Health, in 2000, outlined some of the distinguishing features of autopathography. Namely, it provides patients with an opportunity to tell their stories outside of traditional medical case narratives, which often "stifle" patients' more personal (and fleshed out) narratives. After all, the telling of one's own illness narrative is an opportunity to share information, bond, and help other ill people to navigate their understanding of their bodies as politicized landscapes.[4] In the case of HIV/AIDS, autopathography is an opportunity to reject reductive stigmas and to offer a story that is more truthfully reflective of the moral dilemmas, difficult circumstances, and complications that accompany one's diagnosis and illness.

Chapter One, "Spiritual Hospitality," offers an overview of the facility, which I have called, for the purposes of this book, "The Space." It begins by considering the day-to-day life of residents at this HIV/AIDS facility. I focus on a few residents, detailing their journeys before and after I met them. I also introduce the many factors that differentiate this facility from other skilled nursing facilities, including the average age of residents (forty-five), residents' relationship to drug addiction and prostitution, and the socially, economically, and politically isolating nature of this illness.

Chapter Two, "The Space," centers on the question: How do AIDS patients negotiate self-identity in light of their illness?

Chapter Three, "Seven Lives," looks at the process of negotiating one's illness while being in a community of people at different stages of the same illness.

Chapter Four, "Nine Deaths," continues to narrate this negotiation of illness through the deaths of nine members of our community over the course of two years. Chapter Five, "Losing It," contains my own introspective stories of the emotional and physical challenges that I faced as a caregiver and the challenges

---

4. Aronson, "Autopathography," 1599.

that other caregivers face when trying to provide love and support in the face of ongoing physical suffering and death. Following a consideration of the toll that caregiving takes on the physical and mental state of caregivers, I've included a chapter called "Questions without Answers" (Chapter Six), which focuses on the value of separating the desire to help from the desire to heal; it considers the multifarious opportunities to sit through suffering and turmoil prayerfully rather than being a "praying problem solver."

Finally, in Chapter Seven, the conclusion, I reflect back on my experience of embedding myself in and writing about this community, especially as I experienced it as a "visitor" after my departure. In between the chapters, I include a series of parenthetical chapters—parenthetical stories—to bridge residents' stories with first person narratives.

As previously mentioned, I did not enter The Space as a fieldworker or researcher, or even as a chaplain: I arrived as a volunteer. Because the facility was without a chaplain, I volunteered to be a prayer partner. I was hustling between my life as a professor—where I led discussions about the stories of marginalized people—and going to a place where I listened to all types of stories told from the margins. In African American literature, I saw stories as a way of cautioning us about the cyclical bent of history. The urgency of residents' stories presented an equally valuable opportunity to think about how to memorialize a community that, like the African American community, had been rendered silent, invisible, and unimportant, but on a shorter historical continuum. I often thought about the plethora of black writers we now celebrate—like Zora Neale Hurston, Langston Hughes, and Nella Larsen—who died in obscurity and poverty, only to be resurrected and held in acclaim a generation later. I wanted to be a part of this community's living voice. At no point in my work at The Space did I imagine this would become a book project, but as a career academic, I suppose I am always making inferences and drawing conclusions, even when I'm not conscious of it. More exactly, I was constantly struggling with questions about how the moral stigma attached to

HIV and AIDS was impacting the way the residents reconstructed their lives for an audience.

I have changed the names of all of the residents represented in this book. I have also interchanged some elements of their personalities and habits to further disguise their identity. Therefore, while the physical descriptions, events, and narratives are true, the identifying features of particular residents have been interposed. I kept meticulous journals while I was chaplain and started work on this project five years after I ceased serving, and, to my knowledge, only one of the residents discussed here is still living.

I started doing chaplaincy work straight out of divinity school—without even one day of real-world experience—but prior to that I was trained as an oral historian, folklorist, and ethnographer in my doctoral work, which preceded divinity school. It is essential to note this, because these are the methodologies that influence the way I think about stories and community. According to the Oral History Association, oral history, the oldest form of historical inquiry, refers to traditional methods of collecting, safeguarding, and giving voice to the memories of people and communities. The American Folklore Society defines folklore study somewhat differently. Folklore is "the body of traditional art, literature, knowledge and practice that is disseminated largely through oral communication and behavioral example." Every group shares a body of traditions that can be considered "folklore." Folklore is ethnographic and participatory. It is conducted *where people are*—where they live or where they congregate. Oral history research allows appropriate space for an interpreter (or researcher) to hear and record residents' stories, while folklore is primarily participatory as it is collected.

In folklore, the greater the intimacy in the relationship between the collector and the subject, the more successful the outcome. This is, of course, the antithesis of how most disciplines perceive fieldwork success, and in this sense, ministry (spiritual caregiving) and folklore are kindred spirits. As Robert Ariss notes in his AIDS ethnography titled *Against Death: The Practice of Living with AIDS*, this work is incredibly difficult to engage ethnographically without constantly re-evaluating where bound-aries lie. As Arliss observes,

> At times I wondered if this activity went beyond the
> reasonable bounds allowed an ethnographer. Identities
> slipped, the observer became the participant, and I the
> observed. However, it is these epistemological and onto-
> logical shifts that drive an anthropological perspective.
> Those working in AIDS, whether they be educators, lob-
> byists or bureaucrats also frequently bear more than one
> role or identity. It is not uncommon for individuals to be
> highly conscious of this multiplicity of self.[5]

In addition to speaking to the socio-spiritual dilemmas that are unique to HIV/AIDS, this statement speaks to the reality that many of the hats we wear as academics and caregivers can stand in conflict, and we must engage in self-examination *as humans* to un-ravel these contradictions. These conflicts are often a consequence of the reality that issues facing HIV/AIDS patients will always be vastly different from the problems and concerns facing other chronic or palliative care patients. As one researcher noted, while stigma may be a central factor in the lives of patients with other ill-nesses, "individuals with HIV/AIDS … reported stronger feelings of stigma than the individuals with cancer" and other diseases, a pattern indicating that while the nature of the illness impacts self-perception, the treatment of people with HIV/AIDS by others is generally more devastating than the disease itself.[6] The amount of isolation that people with HIV and AIDS face at the end of their lives has raised unique concerns for medical caregivers, pastoral caregivers, families, and communities. This was particularly acute among ethnic minorities, who made up the vast majority of our clientele, and who negotiated their illness in communities already steeped in social and sexual stigmas. Cathy Cohen accurately notes in *The Boundaries of Blackness* that to address the issue of AIDS in the Black community is to also acknowledge the existence of black male homosexuality and its associated behaviors, and to

5. Ariss, *Against Death*, 7–8.
6. Fife, *Doing Fieldwork*, 63.

determine if these individuals are "worthy" of the time and atten-tion of Black political agendas.[7]

I am an urban, African American woman and identify strong-ly with the historical significations of each of these categories. But beyond these visible categories, I generally avoided discussing my background, my education, or my full-time profession with residents. I found labels like "professor" to provoke distance. The residents called me "Chap," and that's who I was. In my capacity as chaplain serving a unique community, I saw myself as having two roles. First, I wished to let the residents know—through my words and actions—that contrary to anything they may have been led to think or believe in their lives, God does not wish to judge them. God only wishes to love them; this liberates God's perfect love, and our relationship to it, from the flawed conditions in which humans live. Second, I wanted to help people who were dealing with physi-cal or emotional suffering to find a place of peace in their lives. Having them find this peace in Christianity was secondary to me. The "space" within us that is free of judgment and pure in love, and that desires to do no harm, can be called Christian or Buddhist or Jewish or Islamic or Hindu or Sheik, or it can be undesignated—it doesn't matter—so long as, on our journey, we are given access to the gift of peace and spiritual quietude that comes from knowing and spreading our highest expression of love.

In the collaborative memoir that follows, I hope the intersec-tion of the profane and the sacred, perfect peace and persistent disquietude, reveals the ways that this illness brought me to my fullest humanity, and called so many of us—whether we were watching it on the news or living it up close—to think about what it means to live more humanly.

7. Cohen, *The Boundaries of Blackness*, 14.

What you seek is seeking you.

—RUMI

1

Spiritual Hospitality

If someone were to ask me what I remember the most about my five years as an HIV/AIDS chaplain, it would be this:

A thirty-year-old Hispanic male resident named Sam is slowly shuffling across the dining room floor. Nobody knows if Sam was born with a mental disability or if his arrested development is HIV-related, but we all know that Sam doesn't speak much, or make eye contact, or show emotion. In fact, the narrative assigned to Sam is that he never had a family, that he was somehow born of himself, then sucked into a vacuum along with other abandoned particles, then emptied onto the doorstep of The Space. Nothing about him easily disavows this narrative.

So Sam is slowly shuffling, hands by his sides, to the front of the dining room—maybe to get a cup of coffee, or to look for a salt packet—when his pants fall all the way down to his ankles. He is not wearing any underwear. He continues shuffling along, and his gait *pre-* and *post-*pants falling down is exactly the same. I am the chaplain and I, like everyone else, am looking. One woman sounds the alarm that he is half naked, but here's the thing: no one reacts.

People look, or shrug, or gawk, or ignore, but no one is particularly moved by his nakedness. Finally an aid runs over and pulls up his pants. And that quickly, the event is over.

I remember this event because years later, despite the deaths and reincarnations I have witnessed, this was the moment when I did the very least that I could do. This motherless man-child's public humiliation happened while I watched. Years later, Sam would die a quiet death. I would perform his farewell service, and his ashes would be returned to our facility since he had no kin. His ashes would sit on a nurse's shelf for three more years, and when that nurse resigned we would lose track of them. Inasmuch as this story is about the people I served, it is also—selfishly—about me, and my desire to make peace with the wide space between seeing and doing, between hearing narratives and giving agency to people's lived experiences.

That begins with the mundane.

It is seven o'clock in the morning on a brisk, autumn, New England day. The work shift is changing at The Space. Nurses, aides, kitchen staff, and administrators arrive by car, bus, and foot, and everyone is clamoring to "make time." They meet up with the weary night staff, creating a small traffic jam at the time clock: they exchange small talk, but what's really on their minds is the clock, and whether the human traffic will cause them to punch in or out seven minutes late, soliciting a reprimand from the shift supervisor.

It wasn't always this way. Once upon a time the staff drifted in, some late, but most arriving early, because there was an emotional investment. HIV/AIDS staffers wanted to do *this* work, however arduous, demanding, and unpredictable. There was a time when the staff did not fill in a time sheet, and the powers that be trusted that the staff arrived when they said they would.

But in 2005—ten years after the opening of The Space, ten years deeper into the HIV/AIDS crisis—everything had changed. Everyone except administrators punched the clock, and the rush of employees to the time clock was just one of the indicators that the work of HIV/AIDS had transformed from sacrificial first responders engaged in an international human health crisis to the business of chronic care.

One nurse remembers the days when nurses knitted blankets for residents' birthdays, or a kitchen staffer cooked an ailing resident any food that fulfilled the fantasy of their last days. Another nurse remembers taking residents to spend Thanksgiving at her mother's house, or coming to The Space in the middle of the night to bid safe passage to a resident taking her last breath. The urgency of the AIDS crisis (people were certain to die), the isolation of the disease (most residents were without family), and the unique social history of the illness (doctors were befuddled about so many elements of the disease) called for a hands-on, twenty-four-hour commitment from staff—emotionally, if not medically and mentally. Being an AIDS worker was not a job; it was a lifestyle. There was a "type" of person who was drawn to this type of work, and it didn't matter if you were a doctor or a janitor at The Space; if you were there, you were the "type." The staff functioned like a family, sharing information about patients formally and informally, depending on maintenance and security staff who knew residents from the neighborhood to supplement background information.

But then the time clock was installed. It was a blow to the ethos of many caregivers who worked hard because they were trusted to do so. The time clock was a metaphor for the evolution of the illness from the "work of the noble" to the "work of the workers." At the same time, across the nation, a new era in the disease was being ushered in. The declining significance of HIV/AIDS in popular media was evident, and yet the amount of work to be done wasn't decreasing.

From the administration's perspective, there was good reason to introduce this new system. A small core of employees had been abusing the honor system: someone had been seen leaving the building to pick up her children from school without signing out. One staff member, rumor had it, had signed in and then left for the better part of the day, returning in time to sign out in the afternoon. There were resounding questions that governed much of the internal machinery of The Space: How can the administration honor the work of staffers in a way that also assures the best care of residents? How can staffers hold each other accountable in a way that does not compromise a trust-based work environment? Perhaps the real question was how we, as a nation, make the transition from crisis terminal care to chronic care alongside the most stigmatized illness of our time.

The Space is a freestanding burnt-brick building in a New England college town that is also a busy urban enclave. Like many college towns—certainly much like New Brunswick, New Jersey, where I attended college—this town is filled with haves and have-nots, wealthy residents with old money and homeless people who populate the town center. There are also clearly distinguishable college types carrying messenger bags and wearing shorts in the middle of winter, as well as local kids with blue collar jobs.

The Space is located half a block from one of those endlessly long "Main Streets" that run from one town to another, intermittently peppered with Dunkin' Donuts and gas stations; Main Street in "town A" is littered with used car dealerships and pawn shops, while Main Street in "town B" is bordered by cafés and boutiques. The Space sits on the borderline between these two polar opposite towns and is jammed between an aging theatrical warehouse on one side and a truck depot on the other. Ironically, The Space is best described as nondescript: it still looks every bit like the factory it was intended to be, with a row of small institution windows that are low-set and uninteresting. Only a row of metallic red ribbons lining the staircase—and in the spring a bundle of chrysanthemums—disrupts the anonymity.

The vast majority of the people who occupy this facility fit a particular profile: most are urban people of color who are struggling with addiction, and most acquired the virus either through intravenous drug use or heterosexual sex. The average resident is modestly educated, possessing a partial or full high school education. Some come to this facility for a "tune-up"—medical management after having strayed from their medication regimen—and they will leave the facility after a three- to six-month stay to resume life on their own. Some, however, come at the end of life, and others wind up staying for years. The average age of residents while I was chaplain was forty-five.

I would characterize the typical resident as having been brought up in some religious tradition, often associated with nationality and experienced primarily through the observation of holidays, eating habits, or other social habits: one respected its "place," but it did not necessarily center one's lived experience. In light of this, I defined myself as a Christian chaplain who advanced the belief that religious traditions are in constant conversation with each other about the reality that the only path to knowledge is suffering, and the only path through suffering is the light, and the light—whoever its messenger—is truth. The guiding principles of all the world's faith traditions promised love, forgiveness, understanding, and peace, a disease that challenged everything we know about being human notwithstanding.

The first year that the national medical community dealt with the AIDS crisis is sometimes referred to as the "medieval period." It raised a new question for medical practitioners that could not be easily answered, specifically, *If I cannot cure, then what am I?* [1]

The quality that distinguished AIDS deaths from other illnesses was its rapidity, specifically the devastatingly short incubation period between infection, full-blown AIDS, and death.

In many ways it was the rapidity that necessitated the shift from "cure" to "care" in dealing with people dying of AIDS. Care included issues that were previously peripheral considerations, including sensitization to the stigmatization of this disease, a sociological re-orientation on the part of medical caregivers. [2] Dr. William Owen, a gay physician who treated many HIV-positive patients during the start of the AIDS epidemic, states,

> I wasn't afraid of getting it from my patients directly. I never used gloves, for instance. Seeing patients with this disease . . . made me, as a gay man, aware of the fact that this disease was probably one of the worst possible things

1. Bayer, *AIDS Doctors*, 63.
2. Ibid., 73.

that could happen to people who were still young ... [It] made me aware of my own vulnerability.[3]

At the root of every conversation about AIDS were social beliefs and behavioral implications. In *AIDS, Identity and Community*, Theo M. Sandfort argues that social attitudes about who gets infected affect the way society in general, and the government in particular, responds to the needs of the infected and the potential victims: in other words, preventive programs among the poor and gay and lesbian communities have been less aggressive than the care for those already infected. In the context of transmittable diseases, this seems to be a counterintuitive approach. Sandfort states, "Societal rejection of homosexuality ... exerts [a] complex influence on HIV prevention. Living in a society that rejects homosexuality, whether in obvious or subtle ways, affects the health status of homosexual people."[4] In Ireland, for example, where Victorian legislation made male homosexual activity a criminal offense, and this offense remained on the statute books, AIDS prevention campaigns that explicitly advocated "safe sex" practices for homosexuals could be construed as condoning criminal behavior.[5]

As a result of the contradictory conditions governing the treatment of gay men with HIV and AIDS, the second population affected by the AIDS epidemic—poor and urban women, many of whom are women of color and women struggling with addiction—were left without community support or acknowledgment of their vulnerability to the disease. As Cathy Cohen notes, "Issues of stigma, fear, rejection, invisibility, classism, sexism, homophobia and drug phobia" all create the boundaries against which the black community constructs a moral and political response to AIDS.[6] As Meredith, a thirty-three-year-old heterosexual mother of two notes,

3. Ibid., 79.
4. Herek, *AIDS, Identity and Community*, 33, 34.
5. Edgar, *AIDS*, 23.
6. Cohen, *The Boundaries of Blackness*, 8.

> If I tell you I was diagnosed with a terminal illness, the normal reaction is "Oh, do you need anything?" ... If I say I have AIDS, the first question is "How did you get it? What have you been doing?" Nobody cares that I am sick, that I hurt, that I am tired all the time. Hey, nobody told me about AIDS! What is my crime? [7]

Given the social stigmas associated with AIDS, end-of-life care had to undergo a shift in consciousness that addressed the competing dilemmas of dealing with outcast communities, an incurable disease, and patients who were often considered "marginally important" prior to their exposure. In what is called the "cultural communication process," it will be essential that members of these communities who are infected become the nexus of inner city sex education campaigns if other members of their communities are to be reached. Just as heterosexual, middle-class women (for example) would not respond to AIDS awareness campaigns designed for gay men, similarly, members of newer high-risk communities are isolated from educational methods that appear to be outside the lens of their experiences.

Rather than offer false hope, end-of-life care for AIDS patients has dealt with the reality that "normal stigma" is an oxymoron that invites social and political re-education. Spiritual caregivers who work with people with HIV/AIDS are political agents, challenging norms from religious, social, sexual, and economic positions.

And even when individual congregations reject the needs of stigmatized bodies, the marginalized individuals, after a lifetime of religious ritual or habit, are beneficiaries of the cultural memory of spiritual hospitality, and its potential beyond a house of worship.

This notion—this openness to spiritual hospitality—was the beginning of this journey.

7. Fee, *AIDS*, 2

(Chapter 1.5)

But before I go further, here's a story about me.

Before I became a chaplain, when I was struggling with my father's illness and impending death, all alone in a new city without a single friend, my boyfriend of three years, who was living and working in another state, ended our relationship without words. I received a package in the mail one day, and when I opened it, a rather expensive gift I'd given him had been packaged and returned to me with a note that said, "This is expensive. You should keep it." And that was it. No explanation, no warning, no words to lend understanding. The irony may have been lost on him that the gift was monogrammed, so he was regifting to me the privilege of having his name inscribed in gold in my home. I put on my coat, walked down the three flights of stairs, and threw it in the dumpster belonging to the Chinese restaurant behind my building.

That expensive gift lying at the bottom of a pile of waste bore witness to the death of a season, and I struggled with why I'd invested so much time in something as fragile as a single union, something that—unlike a movement, or an ideal, or justice—couldn't possibly result in a predictable outcome, or a universal good, or social change. Moreover, what did I expect to get from the relationship? I didn't want to be married (marriage was an institution fraught with too many incurable inequalities for women—even the most devoted of wives knew *that)* and here I was feeling even more empty, alone, and purposeless than ever, all because of a solitary, embarrassingly ordinary human. This void ultimately drew me deeper into the spiritual questioning that had persisted through my Catholic roots, then through my Baptist rebirth in graduate school, and up to my present state as a member of the United Church of Christ.

A few weeks into this questioning, I decided that I needed a change of scenery. I had recently completed my doctorate, and like most recent graduates, I had serious school debt. I was only two years into my first professional job and I had no money, no time, and no energy. But this romantic juggernaut became an occasion to think about what I really wanted to do with my life going forward, and I was keenly aware that having the emotional space to think about this was itself a mercy and a luxury. I booked a flight to see cousins in England, and among the things I packed in my suitcase was a divinity school application.

For the next few weeks, I journaled by the canals in Canterbury. On New Year's Eve, I sat on a metal chair holding a paper cup of soda while an inebriated uncle snoozed right through midnight at a house party in Wembley. I ate fish and chips at Piccadilly Circus, and sipped colorful cocktails with cousins in the West End, hoping all the while that my credit card wouldn't be declined. Then, tucked into a nook of my elderly aunt's sewing room in London, I took to bed and spent a few days working on my divinity school application, hoping that the meaning of life would come to me through the process of answering questions of faith. My aunt, having no idea what would keep an American girl so busy all day and night, brought me big bowls of oatmeal and coffee and biscuits, despite my insistence that I was okay. Her spirit, she said, told her I was doing important work.

An acceptance letter came upon my return to the States.

The following semester, my journey—which left very little space for marinating in sad thoughts—started. During the day I would teach. In the evening, I would drive two and a half hours from Massachusetts to Connecticut to attend divinity school classes. On weekends I would grade papers, then write papers. Having no spare time, I put my grieving on hold for a long, long time.

It is astounding: the great wars and immortal music, the shifted trajectories, the lives ended—and begun—the art that is inspired, or destroyed, all in the name of love. In this regard, the path that led me to The Space is, perhaps, the most normal human story ever told. Love. And yet no story that leads to HIV and AIDS narratives is ordinary. Or absent of love.

The wound is the place where the Light enters you.

—RUMI

2

The Space

Before The Space was a skilled nursing facility, it was the Sunbeam Dress Company, a one-story building about six hundred feet off a busy street. In 1968, the factory made women's clothing in an expansive, nondescript, and dimly lit warehouse—a stark contrast to the smart and modish garments it produced. Like most New England factories, it employed moderately skilled local women who spent their days standing alongside rows of dressmaking tables. Above them, elongated pipe-like rods that were bolted to the ceiling held fluorescent lights above the worktables, providing generous amounts of light for fine stitching. One can only imagine that it was noisy; that the workers were held to a rigorous production schedule; that the glimmer of sunlight that broke through the small high-set windows was an understated novelty.

Then, as now, it was a workingman's town on the one hand, and the home to a high-minded, intellectual class (and university) on the other. There were factories of all kinds: clock factories and gun factories, cheese factories and toy train factories. Working folks, mostly immigrants, paid their taxes, minded their business, and thanked their lucky stars if they had a skill to sell in the competitive labor market.

But shortly after Sunbeam was in full operation, the city—like so many New England towns in the 1970s—undertook a massive redevelopment effort to disassemble the "factory feel" of the town. In the dawn of a new era, *this* New England city would become more livable, more neighborhood-friendly—an attractive settling place that would lure other New Englanders into its borders. With the city seeking to demolish a number of factory eyesores, and with the export of dressmaking to more cheaply run factories, Sunbeam could not compete. The dress factory abandoned shop.

But the Main Street building escaped demolition. In fact, it was temporarily forgotten altogether until, in 1974, it was refurbished, and re-opened by the Fire-lite Company—the makers of industrial alarm systems. When they left the building after sixteen years (they had outgrown the location, but continue to thrive to this day), it remained empty for four years.

Like all New England towns, this town was subject to the ebbs and flows of history: it thrived when the economy was strong and declined during recessions. The locals lived one life; the transient college kids, on a four-year tour of the city, came and went, perhaps oblivious to the reality that life went on after they departed.

In the 1970s, drugs ravaged what was left of the faltering "downtown." To hear some locals tell it, integration was the thing that ravaged the town center, but black and white professionals fled the city for life in the suburbs, leaving white ethnics and the black working poor in gutted neighborhoods. In the 1980s, the AIDS epidemic was added to the woes inflicted on a city in sharp decline.

The first cases of an unnamed, opportunistic, and horrifyingly deadly "cancer" emerged among gay men in nearby New York and in California in the 1980s. The discovery of a virus called HIV was made soon after. By the late 1980s a new group was rivaling gay men as the primary victims of HIV and AIDS: intravenous drug users. In 1986, Jon Parker, a New Englander who was a former injection drug user, was earning his master's degree in public health at Yale University when he decided to venture back to the streets to talk to intravenous drug users about their needs. At one such meeting in Boston, a user brought Jon seven sterile syringes to share with others, inspiring Parker to begin distributing—and later exchanging—needles and syringes on the streets of New Haven and Boston.[1]

With Parker's help, and the help of other advocates of needle exchanges, The Needle Exchange Program Law was passed by a 3-to-1 margin in the Connecticut legislature in early 1990. By November of 1990, needle exchange services were up and running out of a humble but, for many, invaluable mobile van service. They serviced 242 clients initially, and of the 1241 needles distributed, 32.3 percent were returned, in addition to 659 returned "street needles" that had not been distributed through the program.[2]

In the interim, a young woman named Kat relocated to New England from Great Britain; she was married to a history professor, and despite the social and economic comfort that defined her American experience, she was discomforted by the impact that the national AIDS crisis was having on her local community. Determined to do something about the increasing number of local AIDS victims, she began an investigation into the creation of a skilled nursing facility for the treatment of people with AIDS. Harvard Business School undertook her proposed project as a case study. In 1995, her vision was realized in the former location of the Sunbeam Dress factory. The Space became one of only a few nursing facilities in the country providing skilled, inpatient nursing care exclusively for people with HIV and AIDS.

During the first days of opening, the staff cared for a single patient.

This is The Space now: As you enter the front door   a sign reads, "If you are suffering with a cold or flu, please visit us another time." It is *risk*—however nominal, however slight—that greets visitors at the door. Past the entrance is a security desk

1. Lane, "Needle Exchange," 2.

2. Kaplan and Heimer, "Evaluating the New Haven Needle Exchange Program," 7.

with a sliding glass divider. It is generally open. Rows of bright fluorescent lighting in the former Sunbeam Dress Company cast unforgiving light on a long hallway of worn carpeting. The facility is clearly clean (notwithstanding the occasional smell of urine that mixes with the scent of coffee in the early morning) but profoundly tired: the faded pink walls are accessorized by pictures of past residents, many of whom are also *passed* residents—and many of the photographs are yellowed and crooked. As you look at the photographs on the wall, you have a vague sense that the people in them are dead, but of course you cannot pinpoint what provoked this conclusion.

Considering the lackluster brick exterior of The Space, the biggest surprise comes fifty or so feet down a broad hallway: the main dining room is a large, cheery, bright, and welcoming space with a glass roof, pastel floral chairs, cafeteria-style tables, and lots of well-cared-for, happy plants. Off to the left side of the dining room is a weathered piano. To the right is the nurses' station, where The Space transforms from what could be a community center or assisted living facility, into a skilled medical care facility. The transition from comfortable recreation space to nurses' station is smooth, except for the pacing of nurses and nurses' aides—in white lab coats and scrubs decorated with pastel-colored cartoon characters—who are standing, sitting, writing, chatting, and distributing drug cocktails.

At The Space, every resident must dress and go to the dining room for breakfast at eight. Residents are told that they will be sent back to their rooms if they arrive at the dining room in pajamas, but it's not a threat that is carried out. Almost every morning a handful of residents are in pajamas, and a couple more are missing altogether when breakfast is served. Missing residents are paged by first name on the intercom system (the page echoes throughout the halls and into every room) until they come to the dining room. If they don't appear after several calls, a nurse's aide is dispatched to their rooms to look for them.

Each resident has an assigned seat in the dining room. Breakfast is usually some combination of toast, sausages, eggs, oatmeal, and pancakes. Fresh fruit is generally served on the side, and generally abandoned. The dietician, a former apprentice at the New Orleans Ritz Carlton, is a miracle worker with a handful of ingredients and a whisk. After breakfast, residents fill their travel mugs with coffee or tea from a community hot beverage station; then they make their way to the back patio for a cigarette.

Smoking is a persistent and unsolvable problem in this community. Only three to seven percent of all Americans who try to quit smoking every year succeed; being among this number is even less likely when considering a history of drug addiction. To say that the business of smoking governs almost every waking hour at The Space—*When can I smoke? How much can I smoke? How do I get cigarettes (with or without money and transportation to a store)?*— is understating the obsession most residents have with smoking and smoking-related issues. Group smoking times, which mainly take place on the facility's rear deck, are the primary social events, and residents relish what they believe to be the "medicinal" effects of smoking. Many reported that cigarettes relax them, calm "the shakes," help their digestion, and even ease bowel movements.

But smoking, a troublesome addiction in general, is more problematic in a medical setting for a number of reasons. Many residents, after taking their daily cocktail each morning, are prone to dozing, and on a few occasions residents have burned holes through coat sleeves or pant legs with their cigarettes. Moreover, residents who are room-bound have been known to sneak a cigarette out an open window. They rarely get away with this, as the smoke quickly seeps through the vents and doors. Sores and infections of the mouth, tongue, and lips, as well as mouth cancers, are all potential consequences of long-term smoking with HIV. And while HIV medications strengthen immunity, smoking generally weakens it, thus countering the effects of some medications, and leaving patients vulnerable to a plethora of other ailments. What's more, increased risk of emphysema, heart and blood flow problems, greater HPV risk, and smoke damage to already compromised kidneys, liver, and bladder are just some of the life-compromising consequences of smoking with HIV. Still, cigarettes are as revered among this population as gold. According to the New York State Department of Health AIDS Institute, while HIV is a manageable chronic disease, 50 to 70 percent of people with HIV are cigarette smokers, a number that represents as much as triple the smoking rate of the general population.[3] The bottom line is that smoking arrests healing. When I met Laura, a recovering drug addict who was a long-term resident at The Space, she had been struggling with persistent infections in her left foot, and she was informed that a partial amputation would be necessary. Laura had been confined to a wheelchair for many years and her paralysis was irreversible; nevertheless, the idea of losing her foot affirmed the demise of mobility. Prior to the news of her amputation, she held out hope beyond any medical actuality that if she followed all of her doctor's directions, went to occupational therapy, and took her meds, she might walk again some day. On the day I visited her in the hospital pre-amputation, a doctor informed her quite plainly that there was a certain futility in performing such a surgery when her excessive smoking (a pack and a half a day) would thwart her body's efforts to heal. She responded resolutely that she had decided she would not give up her foot, nor would she give up her cigarettes, *for anything*. However legal the distribution of cigarettes, the unfortunate reality is that nicotine is a mood-altering, addictive drug. As one source notes, condoning nicotine use for a drug addict is almost like telling an alcoholic to give up rum, scotch, and whiskey, but not beer.

After breakfast and a morning cigarette, residents either retire to their rooms to watch television and nap, or they congregate in the recreation area, where they watch television and talk or work on ongoing craft projects (watercolor projects and coloring books are popular and left within reach). Residents have various levels of mobility and represent every stage of illness, from full agility to palliative care. A variety of support groups are scheduled throughout the day, including recovery groups, grief and loss groups, life skills classes, and men and women's groups. There are

3. New York State Department of Health AIDS Institute, "HIV and Smoking," 5.

also art classes, exercise classes and meditation classes, nutritional information classes, and even a cooking group. Many residents participate in regular community-wide bingo games, where they earn pretend money to buy real items, including toiletries, socks, or snacks. Days out, organized by the two-person recreation department, include shopping trips, fishing excursions, and outings to movies, local concerts, fairs, and carnivals. In the sense that they keep people's spirits up and keep residents optimistic and connected to the community, the recreation department is the lifeline of The Space. Residents can request any type of activity, and it is likely to be realized. One year, a full spa experience was created for the residents in the art room, complete with manicures, pedicures, facials, shoulder massages, and head rubs. The spa "clients" passed through organza drapes, listened to classical music, and sipped tea while they waited. Residents without "appointments" were directed to an area where they received neck massages while they waited. It was clear that the recreation director and assistant director enjoyed the realization of such creative fantasies as much as the residents did and took the work of emotional reprieve very seriously.

Visiting groups of volunteers provide other forms of entertainment, including live bands, magicians, dance performances by spiritual groups, and choirs. A few times a year a DJ comes in, and the dining room is transformed into a nightclub. Residents are also able to attend outside support groups, such as Alcoholics Anonymous or Narcotics Anonymous meetings, or church services.

Lunch is served at twelve-thirty and includes a standard choice of a deli sandwich or hamburger, potato salad or French fries, and fruit or yogurt. In addition to these "standard" choices, residents can opt for a number of special meals. Watching the residents partake in meals was a lesson for me in the futility of preaching about waste. On some days, when I had long shifts, my mouth would water as I passed the dining room and watched a resident picking over a sloppy Joe and pushing aside an apple. "That looks just delicious," I would say. "It's okay," was the usual response. Or, "It's the same ole thing . . . ." It is not unusual to see fruit, milk, and other healthy choices left on the plates. Once these healthy options are served on a resident's tray in the dining room, they cannot be given to another resident. They must, then, be thrown away. The amount of daily waste is astounding and a constant source of concern for the facility's head chef.

By three o'clock there are rumblings. Residents are beginning to get restless and hungry. The three o'clock snack is usually a sandwich or an ice cream cup and juice, or all three if the resident wishes. Residents are not allowed to have food in their rooms, but since snacks are not served in the dining room (they are passed out at the room entrance) it is inevitable that food will be consumed, or stored, or—worst of all—forgotten in a dresser drawer or on a shelf.

Dinner, which is served at six-thirty, is followed at nine o'clock by a bedtime snack. In between, residents can request food from the nurses' station or purchase a snack from a vending machine in the common area. It is also not unusual for mobile residents to do "store runs" and return with chips, cookies, and other "unapproved" treats. Sometimes, late at night, residents will order disallowed meals, like Chinese takeout or pizza.

Despite the bustle of activity, boredom is a serious problem at The Space, and it resembles a senior nursing facility in this way. There is a lot of sitting and watching people and doing nothing—this among a population of fairly young people. One resident named Joe spends most the day sitting in his wheelchair in the hallway closest to the nurses' station watching people pass. A few people may stop and say hello to him, and he will respond in kind, but the conversation rarely goes any further. No one knows (or asks) much about Joe—his interests, his likes or dislikes, or anything that would lend insight into what you might say to him beyond "hello." When there are no passersby, he plays with his fingers with great interest, or picks his nose impulsively, or takes a little nap. Sometimes he looks around at nothing in particular. What's odd about Joe to someone like me, a chaplain without medical or in-depth training in mental infirmities, is that he seems to be waiting to be engaged, but once he receives engagement, he becomes unresponsive. Here is a typical exchange between Joe and me one morning, when he seemed to be beckoning me over:

"Good morning, Joe."

"Yup," he waved in my direction.

"How are you today?" (I know that I sounded overly cheery, like a beauty pageant contestant.)

"Okay-ye-guess," he looked away from me.

"Did you sleep well last night?"

"Yup," he scratched his head.

"Good! And how was breakfast this morning?"

"Okay-ye-guess," he looked past me. I think he was looking at a painting on the wall.

"Joe, would you like me to pray with you this morning?"

He picked his nose with swift deliberateness then said, almost in a tone of surrender, "Okay-ye-guess."

I looked at his fingers, which had just left his nose, then took both of his hands in mine and prayed with him. As soon as I walked away his expression looked as if he was summoning me back, as if he had forgotten to tell me something. He hadn't.

Another resident, named Lopez, spends all day in bed. Lopez is a forty-five-year old Puerto Rican man who was transferred to The Space from prison, and he has found a way to get and smoke marijuana in bed everyday. The nurses smell it, but can never find it, and security guards have searched his room many times to no avail. He claims he is too sick and too nauseated to come to the dining room for meals. His room is an unsanitary mess, and it is difficult to navigate a path from the doorway to his bed when I visit. Three times a day he pulls on his oversized pants and, holding them up, makes his way down the long hallway to the gazebo, where he chain-smokes in silence for a while before returning to his bed.

In many cases, a life-long battle with drug addiction and associated behavior (such as hustling or prostitution) has caused residents, like Lopez, to become isolated from their families. In this HIV-positive community, residents are the second or third generation to live in poverty, facing joblessness, poor schools, inadequate housing, and few opportunities to climb out of destitution—particularly since many are addicts, and have been in the pipeline from prison to HIV in-facility care. Approximately 80 percent of America's inmates—1.8 million—were either high at the time of their crimes, committed their offenses to get money to buy drugs, have a history of alcohol or drug abuse and addiction, or share some mix of these characteristics. It is difficult to parse incarceration histories from drug-related crimes or drug addiction histories; what is clear is that all three are a part of many residents' HIV stories. According to the Connecticut Department of Public Health, as of December 2015 there were almost 21,000 reported cases of people living with HIV and AIDS in the state of Connecticut, of which 41 percent were intravenous drug users. The largest population of infected people in 2015 were black men between the ages of thirty and thirty-nine, who participated in intravenous drug use.[4]

The relationship between residents and staff is not typical of what you might observe at other nursing facilities, mainly because the average resident is the same age as the average staff member. Therefore, the staff are dealing with residents who are often aware that they are negotiating their needs with their contemporaries. Also many of the staff know the residents from local (and insular) communities.

As chaplain, it was immediately evident to me that there was a difference between the ways nurses indicated to me that someone "wanted" prayer versus someone "needing" prayer. People who "wanted" prayer were those who called for me through the nurses. People who "needed" prayer were usually the people who were prone to cursing and defiance, and the nurses hoped that a visit from the chaplain might "get them some religion."

One nurse described residents as obnoxiously entitled. "You spend your whole life drugging and living on the streets—under some bridge—and now you want me to run when you ring your call bell because you need your meds—*now*? How did you get your

---

4. New York State Department of Health AIDS Institute, "HIV and Smoking," 4.

meds *now* on the streets? They know who they can pull that nonsense with, and who they can't pull it with, and I'm not the one." Another staff member, a woman in food services, noted, "Residents think they are at a hotel—like they are at The Plaza—and we are the maid service. They sit at their lunch table and bark out orders like they've shown up at a restaurant. And some have the nerve to get nasty and curse you out when you don't get them what they want, when they want it."

Residents respond to these claims by reminding me, and others, that depending on the staff for basic care and food, while dealing with illness and addiction—to say nothing of implicit biases based on race, gender, the burden of addiction, and class—is demoralizing and painful.

It is contradictory but true that while every resident at The Space has eerily similar stories, each situation is startlingly unique. There were social workers and teachers who arrived as residents. There were truck drivers and seamstresses, a dancer and a hairdresser. Some had not finished primary school, others had degrees from Yale, Boston University, and UCLA. Some worked toward their GEDs while at The Space. One constant truism is that the vast majority of residents were the second or third generation to live in poverty. The difference between their parents' generation and their own is AIDS.

If The Space had to be big enough to harbor the stories of all the residents—those spoken and those unspoken—it would have to be as large as the city that hosts it. Moreover, if this book were to record all of the life paths that brought residents to their diagnoses with HIV/AIDS and to their residency at The Space, all the pages ever written about AIDS couldn't contain it.

Take, as a first example, Shine.

Shine was raised by her single mother in a working-class New England town. She was a quiet, fair-skinned Italian child with huge black eyes and thick blonde hair. One day, her mother brought home a drug-abusing boyfriend who had become homeless. He brought along some bags, some drugs, and his two teenage children—a boy and a girl. Shine was eleven when her mother's boyfriend came to live with them, and their home became a regular gathering place for the alternately unemployed and underemployed boyfriend, and all of his friends. The steady stream of friends drugged and drank heavily and partied loudly. Shine and her mother became increasingly disconnected from each other, and as her mother became more and more desperate to please her new boyfriend and his comrades, Shine's mother graduated from "just drinking" to marijuana. Then heroine. It wasn't long before her mother's boyfriend began "visiting" Shine's room and, Shine says, "messing with me."

By this time, her mother was in too much of a drug- and alcohol-induced haze to act in her daughter's best interest. When Shine eventually raised objections to her mother—and it is likely her mother already knew what was going on—her mother informed her that she was making up malicious lies because she was jealous of the boyfriend's children.

Shine began stealing some of the drugs around the house for her own use: it helped her to deal with her ever increasing anxiety attacks and mounting depression. One day, her mother caught her using drugs and beat her severely. By this time, she had already stopped going to school. She decided to leave home (where her mother's boyfriend's children and some of the boyfriend's friends had essentially become squatters in every room of the house) and "ran away" to an abandoned house across the street. She stayed there for the next few weeks, watching her mother with her mother's new "family" through a broken window and sneaking in to get food and drugs when no one was around. No one seemed to be looking for her.

When she eventually left the neighborhood, she resorted to prostitution to finance her increasing drug habit. She married her pimp, then left him, then married him again. When one of the many beatings she received from him landed her in the emergency room, she received her HIV diagnosis, with, as she remembers it, bland indifference.

I met her twenty years later.

The Shine I knew was a forty-something-year-old woman with glazed-over black eyes and thinning hair that was black and blonde and gray in different areas. She had full rosy lips that were spotted with large white circular sores. The lower half of her right earlobe was missing: she said an earring had been pulled clear through the flesh during a fight with a boyfriend. Shine was heavy-set in places—her face and her belly were fully rounded—and thin in other places, like her arms and calves. She had no fingernails or toenails, a result of years of drug abuse impacting the circulation of blood to her fingers and toes. She was bound to a wheelchair. Her feet were black and blue and heavily swollen, such that the skin had burst and, consequently, remained heavily bandaged. She spent most of the day nodding in and out of sleep.

Shine did not have any family with whom she had remained in touch, except her imprisoned adult son to whom she wrote on a regular basis. Upon entering her room, you would see his responses to her letters: elaborate drawings depicting nude women with devil's horns and tails, impaled on crosses, blood dripping from their lips and vampire fangs visible beneath ominous sneers. "My son is such a talented artist," she would say to me, as I'd gazed around at bare-breasted devils and vampires on crucifixes.

Shine seemed to have nine lives. She would stop breathing, and nurses would sound the alarm; then she would pop up as if she had just been napping. She'd fall flat on her face, with no sign of movement, and when a nurse picked her up, she'd inhale and—upon exhaling—ask for a candy bar. She would receive last rites, distant family members would be called, and then, within a day, she would be removing her own leg bandages and yelling obscenities into the call button.

Shine's room was neatly kept, and on her night table she kept three Bibles neatly stacked and carefully marked in many places. She also had photos of her son bordered in elaborate frilly frames. Her lotions, perfumes, and pens were in neat rows. This profound orderliness of pretty things seemed to stand in disagreement with the satanic images from her son jacketing the walls.

One nurse's aide told me that she was afraid to go in her room: "There is some kind of evil in there" she said, "something that just ain't right."

One day, while Shine was talking to me, she suddenly looked away, and gave directives to a little boy who was not there. The little boy was named Jimmy, and he seemed to be excessively noisy, such that she could not talk over him. "Stop it Jimmy! I can't hear myself think!" She would say. She told me that Jimmy was small, about seven, and blond and rambunctious. He visited her every day.

Another day, Shine asked me to come to her room. Her television had been yanked out of the wall, and the nurse, who arrived shortly thereafter, proceeded to tell her that her phone would be taken away next. Shine confessed that she had been a "bad girl," cursing at the nurses all night while the other patients tried to sleep, and refusing to get up for breakfast. She was, in every sense of the word, on punishment. She then burst into tears, "What am I suppose to do? Doesn't anyone understand that I am dying? I am dying!"

Shine would reach her ninth life soon. So would her son. Her death would come in a few days, on an unseasonably cold and blustery night, just hours before dawn. Death would pull her from the bed and knock her to the cold, linoleum floor, bruising her temple. The nurse, who was once again annoyed by Shine's dramatics, would hear a thump on the floor. After sighing and asking, *What's wrong now?* she would realize that this was not another dress rehearsal for death. She would try to save her. She would eventually look away, realizing that this time is really was too late.

Shine's story was a reminder of the movement of stories from the past to the present and back again. In thinking of the body as a landscape, the physical indicators of her illness told one story and her life narrative offered the story's preface. Both stories—the past and the present body—provoked discomfort. Ultimately, what she could not cure in her body, she could negotiate by retracing her path and seeking understanding. Her attention-seeking, I would argue, was her desire to use words to make her body visible beyond illness.

Another one of the first residents I met when I came to The Space was Shelia, a forty-five-year-old woman who had been in recovery for almost two years.

Shelia was Amazonian; she was five-feet-nine inches tall, with leathery skin, strong hands, and a resolute posture, albeit leaned up against a cane. What I first noticed about Shelia was her romantically African appearance—her rich, dark brown skin, sharp almond-shaped eyes, broad nose, high-set cheekbones, and full lips—and it seemed that she was from a people and a place that viscerally rejected all things Caucasian. Actually, Shelia was from South Carolina. In the two years she spent at The Space, Shelia learned to manage her own medications and took advantage of every support group available. She quit smoking and studied for her GED. She did so well that she was being transferred to a halfway house, after which she hoped to get her own apartment. As a result of multiple strokes, Shelia lost the use of her left arm. With patient dexterity, she learned to use her right hand to tie shoe laces, open containers, and make plastic, beaded jewelry, all of which she wore in a mass around her neck and arms, all at once.

Everyone knew her as the poster girl for The Space, the "proof" that poor, black, former drug-addicted women could live productively with HIV/AIDS. With hopes of making peace with her adult children, she would send them the pamphlets with her strong, certain image plastered on front. Her children—all professionals—never responded. Every week she attended prayer service and prayed faithfully to have her children back in her life, "in, you know, *some* kind of way."

When I was a volunteer, I would do Shelia's hair every two weeks. Shelia had a head of thick, jet-black hair that had no exposure to chemicals of any kind. I would wash, condition, and brush all of the knots with great carefulness. I would part her hair into small sections and massage coconut oil into her scalp, a level of attention that was a welcomed luxury, like a trip to a high-end salon. Section by section I would wind her hair into smooth, shiny twists that fell into a pattern on her neck. We would chat and eat chocolate. By the time I was done—it generally took about an hour and a half—we would both gaze at her transformation in the mirror, and admire the results of our time together.

When I became the chaplain, however, these twisting sessions had to end. Doing hair was frivolous, according my supervisor—a social worker—and it didn't result in an interaction that was "useful." Chaplaincy existed under the auspices of social services, which was a deviation from chaplaincy at all other facilities in the state (it is generally its own department, or part of recreational services). I, of course, understood my supervisor's position. But it was apparent to me that a spiritual caregiver in an unconventional community needed to invite a broad range of bonding occasions, individually and as a community. Yes, it would, perhaps, be inappropriate for a social worker to do hair, but at The Space, a small and intimate environment, it was not unusual for nurses' aides or the folks on the janitorial staff or other caregivers to do hair or nails or a random "makeover," because maintaining residents' mental well-being was connected to physical upkeep and, more broadly, care and self-esteem.

For example, like many black women, Shelia would never cut her hair, because hair, for Sheila, was about image, and worth, and power; she was wedded to the feeling of her hair touching her neck; it felt like wealth, and worthiness. This sparked a series of conversations about blackness and European beauty standards that, I think, were meaningful to Shelia. It also led to several conversations wherein we shared our views on the nature of God. Shelia was interested in God's "whiteness." I shared with her a scene in Alice Walker's novel *The Color Purple* where Celie, the central protagonist, realizes that God is not the old white man in the sky that she had, for so long, imagined him to be. Removing this image allowed her room to become God's image. God, Shelia realized, was something within her, and was her. God was all that she had come through and all she could become. Hair was an entrance point to reimagining the world and renegotiating her sense of self. Indeed, the business of doing hair among black women in residence was far from an exercise in vanity. It was what it has always been for black women: a place to wrestle with identity. It was a practice of relaxation, a show of trust, an expression of common cultural identification, and an opportunity for more intimate conversation.

Around the time that I became chaplain, Shelia was told that she was well enough to leave our skilled nursing facility and live independently. This was good news for Shelia. She talked persistently about her desire to live on her own, to have her own small place where she could cook meals, have friends over (although she did not have any friends that I was aware of), and independently handle her finances. She was matched with a group home, which meant that although she would not be fully independent, she would have significantly more autonomy than she had at The Space. Two weeks before Shelia was to make her transition out of The Space, I snuck her away and did her hair as carefully and neatly as I could. I also requested permission to take her to lunch at a local diner.

As we left the restaurant, it began to snow; still, I agreed to drive into the city so that she could show me her new home. It was a lovely three-story house in a quiet working-class neighborhood, and, with the snow falling on the mint green rafters, I imagined that it was just the type of home she longed for.

After driving around the city we returned to The Space and prayed together. Then I left. The next week she prepared to leave. I had not seen her since our day out and as I arrived on the morning of her departure, I saw her making her way over to me. As she got closer I could see she had a bitter look on her face. "Look what you did," she said.

"What?" I asked.

"Right here!" She held onto a piece of her hair that had come undone. "It's falling apart. You need to do this over."

I looked at her puzzled. "Is that it?" I asked.

"What do you mean?" She looked at me, equally puzzled, still holding the unraveled hair in her hands. "You didn't do it right."

"I won't have time to do that today," I responded dryly. "I have too many people I need to see."

She turned her back to me. "Whatever," she said. I started talking to another resident who was nearby. The other resident then commented, "Did you know that Shelia is leaving us on Monday?"

"Yes," I responded, "I did know that. In fact, we went out to celebrate." I attempted to sound light-hearted. Shelia looked over at me and thought for a second. "You coming back before I leave on Monday so that you can redo this hair?"

"No," I said.

"Okay," she responded. We looked at each other in silence. Then a nurse called me over, and I walked away. I didn't see her for the rest of the day. I left later that afternoon, feeling empathy for her children—for whom I hadn't considered feeling empathy before.

Shelia spent her entire life drifting. She started her "career" as a professional groupie to several seventies bands. Then she graduated to drug use at concerts and after parties that the A-listers didn't go to. She was leaving The Space, but to do what? Born to a drug-addicted mother, turned out to prostitute by her brother, beaten by the only man who ever said "I love you" (which was as true as all the other lies he'd told), Shelia had had few opportunities in life to give or receive respect. The crack pipe was both a noose around her neck and her most valuable charm necklace, and now that it was gone, there was nothing to soften the blow. Was the God I offered her a sustainable opiate?

This incident with Shelia was typical of the type of behavior that, without context, can be read by the clinical staff as insufferable entitlement. But as Susannah B. Mintz notes in *Unruly Bodies: Life Writing by Women with Disabilities*, "These are body stories that suggest how thoroughly impairment, loss of function or unusual body contours matter to a person's sense of self," but not in ways that would speak to a traditional patriarchal negotiation of continuous distress, and certainly not in ways that would speak to mainstream assignments of behavioral patterns.[5]

---

5. Mintz, *Unruly Bodies*, 212.

Three months after she left I saw Shelia, thin and disheveled, sitting at a bus stop, nodding off. I can only assume that she reengaged in drug use and she was dismissed from the group home setting. I wondered if she was homeless again. She looked in my direction, but I couldn't tell if she was looking at me or recognized me. She had long extensions in her hair—they reached her waist and looked like dreadlocks—and she grabbed some hair in a bundle and held it up in my direction. I wasn't sure why, but I smiled in her direction and nodded approvingly.

After that, I never saw Shelia again.

During my first year at The Space, the recreation department hosted a version of "The Dating Game" for Valentine's Day. A forty-five-year-old resident named Laura was asked to describe her idea of a "perfect date." She responded, "I guess going on any date would be perfect. Never had one."

While this may seem unusual, add to it the fact that Laura had been married for more than seven years and had a boyfriend whose tenure in her life overlapped with her marriage. Her boyfriend lived with a woman he claimed was his landlady, but Laura suspected they were involved in a relationship. Since she had never (in five years) seen where he lived, she could not say who the woman *really* was. She knew only that the woman often refused to put her boyfriend on the phone when she called.

"Why do you keep calling here bothering this man?" The woman on the other end would say to Laura. "Anyway, he is not here. And if he was, he wouldn't want to talk to you." Laura assigned no blame to the boyfriend—who came to see her sporadically—nor did she assume the boyfriend was the original author of the message the woman was giving her.

Laura was a dark-skinned woman with incredibly thick glasses that shrunk her eyes by half. She had been confined to a wheelchair for years. The chair was "low-tech," and getting around depended entirely on the strength of her arms. She wore generous amounts of beaded and gold jewelry (necklaces, rings, bracelets, and earrings) and spoke in clear, curt phrases: "I hungry," "What up?" "I'm bored." She was an avid reader of anything she could get her hands on—newspapers, novels, books of poetry—but one wondered if her comprehension level was on par with her proclivity for story consumption.

Laura's boyfriend would sometimes go months without calling her or returning her calls to him, then he would appear at The Space and spend an hour or so with her alone in her room. More confounding than his behavior was her understanding of what a relationship ought to entail, and of whether her current relationship was providing anything to her at all. As she expressed it to anyone who would listen, Laura wanted more and felt she deserved more, but in the absence of "normal" what she had was "enough." In her opinion, it was better than nothing.

And what could anyone do about the four-foot-tall, one-eyed boyfriend who showed up, shut her door, had sex with her motionless lower half, and then left? And what was our place in regulating her admittedly unprotected sex with a boyfriend who, according to her, didn't believe she really had the virus? The fact that he didn't know The Space was an HIV facility speaks to his potential mental limitations.

Laura's story speaks to the dilemmas at the nexus of disability identity, which requires that people with disabilities negotiate alternative means of imaging their wholeness. Sometimes these efforts lead to a panacea (her boyfriend was like a theatrical attempt at playing "normal"); other times disabled people construct a community in which the telling of their own story is validated by others' receptiveness to it. In Laura's case, I think she found the wholeness she was seeking—though not through her romantic relationship. I have watched Laura helping other disabled residents in small acts of courtesy and solidarity: holding doors, sharing stories, comparing mobility progress notes. All of these experiences of community account for what I saw as Laura's genuine experience of recovering esteem.

One of the ways The Space promoted the emotional healing of mentally fractured residents was by focusing attention away from the physical condition and onto personal strengths and abilities. The idea is not to distract residents from thinking about their lives; rather, the idea is to affirm that everyone has gifts, talents, and positive traits that have utility within the community, and which they can nurture in solitude.

An example of this was a resident named Julio who came to The Space with full-blown AIDS and squamous cell carcinoma—mouth cancer. The cancer had eaten away almost the entire right side of his face. Ten years before we met, Julio was a classical guitar player in night clubs in lower Manhattan. He was raised in a small village in Puerto Rico outside of Ponce, where he inherited a love of classical guitar from his grandfather. After coming to the States he dedicated all of his energy to his craft, playing anywhere he could find a "gig"—in bands and at dinner clubs. He also played small venues in and around New York and gave private guitar lessons to supplement his income.

Even after Julio contracted the virus—he started using intravenous drugs with some of his musician friends—he did not curtail his lifestyle, which included late-night sets, early morning day jobs, and composing in the margins. Drugs kept things moving. His complications mounted, and having burned many bridges with both family and friends, to whom he owed, by now, significant amounts of money, he wound up at The Space. When he arrived, he brought with him the only things he hadn't sold or lost: an electric guitar and a handful of family photos.

Julio was extremely weak when he arrived, and due to the advanced state of the cancer in his mouth, he spoke in a muffled tone. His entire face was wrapped in gauze most of the time, and when it wasn't, the nursing staff seemed to be exerting effort to keep him in his room.

As a teenager, I'd taken guitar lessons, and I'd learned as close as I could to nothing in the course of a year. On the day we met, after doing Julio's spiritual assessment, I mentioned that I tried to play the guitar as a teen. For the first time since I'd met him, Julio's eyes lit up. I confessed that I'd learned very little and share my music lesson stories with him. It was the first time a resident seemed interested in listening to me tell stories; perhaps it was a welcomed distraction from his own debilitating pain.

"Maybe I'll bring my guitar one day and you can teach me something," I suggested. Julio came to life.

I started bringing my guitar on a regular basis. I would sit in his room—he in his bed—each of us holding our respective instruments. At first, he tried to get a sense of what I knew, and he discovered the answer to that was "little to nothing." He started trying to teach me a few basic chords. In his existence at The Space, Julio was quiet, withdrawn, depressed, and in pain. But when he picked up his guitar for our lessons, he was animated, funny, and sarcastic. A few weeks in he said to me, "I don't know how to say this, but maybe you are hopeless. Still, we play." I picked up my guitar knowing that he was right. I was not a musician, but this was—so far—the most rewarding musical experience of my life.

Little by little, Julio deteriorated. One day he said to me, "Play whatever you can. I'll listen today." He nodded his head along to the off-key chords I played with enthusiasm. I was leaving in a few days to study Indian religion in Hawaii, and I didn't think we had much time left together.

"Julio," I said to him before I left, "I am going far away to study for a while. Two months. I will miss you, but I will see you when I get back." He looked sad at first, then pained. "You go, Chap. You have fun for both of us." He didn't say he would see me when I returned.

"Take my guitar," he said. "You can have it."

"No, no," I said. "You'll need it. But I will play it for you when I get back." He rolled his eyes animatedly. "Aye!" he said, and drifted off to sleep. The doctors told me that he would not be alive when I returned.

I thought of Julio often while I was away, and called weekly to check on him. "He's hanging in there," the nurses would say. "No better, no worse."

"Well, tell him I called," I'd request. Seven weeks passed. I continued to call to check on him and other patients.

"You know," said the nurse, "I give Julio all of your messages and it's the one time I see him smile. I believe that man is waiting for you."

The following week I returned and went straight to see Julio. He was slumped in the bed barely awake, and his face was now completely bandaged to cover the growing deformity. He was in intense pain.

"Hello, my friend," I said.

He smiled. "I missed your bad playing. Play for me, will you?" I picked up his guitar and plucked out an awful tune.

"That's good," he said, "very good." As he drifted off to sleep, I left his room to catch up with a host of other residents. I didn't arrive home until late that night.

Around midnight The Space called. Julio had just passed away peacefully.

Out beyond ideas of wrongdoing and right doing there is a field.
I'll meet you there.

—RUMI

3

Seven Lives

A woman named Jeanie arrived at The Space under the cloak of night. This hiding—this irremovable veil, this shadowy sojourning—was only the subtext of her story. Imagine: the man who allegedly raped her and infected her with the virus was also a resident at The Space, yet the shame and the seemingly obligatory evasiveness were her cross to bear entirely. During her first few days, I saw her peeking around corners fretfully and tiptoeing dubiously. As the days went by, she took to sitting in a corner of the recreation room kneading her hands and biting her lower lip until a permanent crease appeared in her flesh.

Jeanie was a slender forty-five-year-old black woman with a short neat Afro framing her caramel-colored skin. She had large, oval, skeptical eyes. She smiled easily, but withdrew her smile just as quickly. Her family—which included her two adult children and her sister—had met with the staff and expressed their concern about her mental stability while living at the same facility as her attacker. He was never convicted of sexually assaulting Jeanie, and it is unclear how well acquainted the two were, if at all, before the incident. Her family was afraid that the stress of being around her accuser would exacerbate her existing health problems.

I'm taking no liberties here when I suggest that no one who had interacted with her accuser—no one—would doubt the possibility that he was guilty. The accused, Lyndon, had spent almost two decades in jail for other crimes. He was now a sixty-year-old man. Though confined to a wheelchair, he was quite strapping—broad and bulky—and standing, I can only imagine, he would have been well over six feet five inches tall. Lyndon often gripped the side of his wheelchair as though he was preparing to rise up, but he never did He smiled occasionally if, say, his favorite team wins a game, but his smile seemed to exaggerate the emptiness of his stare.

Lyndon wasn't always so neutral, it seems. Many years ago a fight with one of his prostitutes—who also happened to be his girlfriend—ended with him chasing her out of their apartment and stabbing her repeatedly, mortally wounding her in broad daylight. And that was what we saw, or chose to see, in him: the soullessness of his empty stare, the reality of his past. Like Jeanie, we marinated in it. In the years I'd known him, he'd never had a visitor—save the volunteers who stopped by to play chess—and he seemed indifferent to friendlessness, too. On holidays, when others entertained guests, he watched from the sidelines expressing neither sadness nor glee.

One day a nurse told me that Lyndon's mother had died in Georgia, and I was asked to inform him of her death. Of all of the residents at The Space, Lyndon was the only one I talked to at arm's length. I'd heard tales about his life as a pimp and his merciless distribution of punishment to anyone who dared to cross him. And I'd seen for myself his muted response to everything around him—including the death of fellow residents. I entered his room reservedly.

"Good morning, Lyndon," I began.

"Yup."

"I'm afraid I have some bad news to share with you this morning. It's about your mother. We received a call this morning telling us that she—she passed last night, Lyndon."

"Umph."

"I'm deeply, deeply sorry. Is there anything that I can do—any calls that you'd like me to make?"

"Nope." His expression remained unchanged, except for the slightest trace of a grin in the corners of his mouth. He stared steadily at the television.

"Okay. I'd be happy to pray with you now—or another time if you'd like."

"Yup."

"Now? Would you like me to pray with you now?"

"Nope. 'Nother time, Hmm-mm."

With a few more words of comfort, I took leave of his room, and a cold air seemed to usher me out.

Within a few weeks of his mother passing, it was determined that The Space was no longer a suitable facility for Lyndon. His viral load was undetectable; therefore, he was essentially too well to retain residency, but too incapacitated to be sent back to prison. It took a few months to find another facility for him, given his HIV status, his history of violent crime, and his psychological limitations. He responded to the news that he would be transferred with the same muted affect he had demonstrated during his tenure at The Space. And soon enough, he was gone, but not before Jeanie, intimidated and vulnerable, left.

A year passed, and while Lyndon's absence allowed some to breathe more easily at first—especially the nurses' aides who were regularly cursed out by Lyndon—other "Lyndons" came.

For example, like a hurricane of irrepressible, anxious energy, Steven-from-The-Bronx arrived. Steven was an old-fashioned loud-mouth who talked on and on about "the joint" and the value of "getting ovah it"—whatever "it" was. *You got the virus? Get ovah it. You infected your girl? Get ovah it. You play, you pay. And at least you ain't in the joint.*

Steven was transferred straight out of his prison room to The Space. He referred to his room in prison terms. Steven would call down to the nurses, "Can you bring pudding to cell 14?" and they would remind him that he was in "room" 14. His declarations were delivered in a decisive and boisterous manner, and he'd throw in an off-handed shrug for good measure. *Yeah, I'll have coffee* (shrug); *I didn't take my meds today* (shrug); *I got a shit-load of cigarettes stashed under my bed* (shrug); *You're dying?* (shrug), *get ovah it.*

One day Steven decided to attend a "grief and loss group" I had organized at the residents' request. After taking a seat, he proceeded to tell a resident who had infected his wife and child—both of whom had subsequently died from the virus--that he needed to "get ovah it."

"You're still here, right?" he shrugged, "So move it along, buddy." He crossed his arms and sat back in his chair, satisfied. Then, for emphasis, "Just move it along, brother."

"The purpose of this group," I reminded him, "is to do just what we were doing: to process grief and to talk about our losses."

"You ever been in the joint, sister?" he leaned forward in his chair and pointed at me. "Let me tell you something. This place is a freakin' country club compared to the joint." He turned his pointing finger to the grieving man. "He should be happy to be here."

Then Steven slumped back in his chair, satisfied with himself once again.

There was something oddly palatable about Steven. Perhaps it was his plainspokenness—his heavy-tongued, no-nonsense candor—that reminded me of people I knew growing up in the Bronx. Perhaps it was that he doggedly simplified problems that were never simple, which allowed us to imagine, for a moment, that they might be.

Two weeks later, Steven woke up one morning, ate his breakfast, put on his coat and hat and walked out the front door. He never came back. A week after that he was found in a crack house. He had died. Someone told us he'd said that he had a good enough life, and that it's good to know when to go.

It struck me that Steven was invested in cutting off stories. One of the ways he dealt with his illness was by asserting that illness is given agency through storytelling. By arresting the narrative process, perhaps Steven imagined himself as disempowering the disease itself. For other residents, however, Steven's attempts to silence them was colonizing, an exercise in social control.

For better or worse, after Steven's departure all was quiet for a season. I settled into running my groups and doing individual prayer with residents. I worked to track down family members who had been lost amid prison stays and drug binges. Along the way I was informed that I was not allowed to sit in the dining room with residents and that that was considered "socializing," not caregiving. When the nurses assured me that there were no health concerns related to a chaplain eating with residents, I resumed my lunches with them and decided to wait for the reprimand. There were innumerable innocuous social interactions that were forbidden; it seemed prohibitions were implemented to discourage staff from being manipulated by the residents, which also presumed a "carryover" of street or prison culture into The Space. The patient-caregiver divisions that were handed down from social services were not based on medical compliance issues and were marginally attentive to prescriptive models used at comparable facilities. The rules were arbitrary, regressive, and segregationist. I knew that I was becoming a bit of a rebel—bucking the de facto dress code by wearing jeans, visiting residents outside of my "billable" hours, and heavy-handedly advocating for residents who weren't being heard. I knew what a fundamental mistake it was to align myself with the residents in a way that isolated me from some administrators. But I was developing my own narrative of what the residents needed, and some needed me to speak for them and stand beside them as much as they needed me to pray over them.

Eventually we received word that Lyndon's HIV could no longer be controlled by the nursing facility he'd moved to. He was coming back. I wasn't alone in dreading his return, his energy draining the lifeblood of both the residents and the staff. On the day he returned, I was walking toward the entrance when I noticed a wheelchair-bound resident waving at me wildly. "Hey, Audrey! Audrey! It's me!" As I got closer I saw Lyndon's large hands gesturing in my direction. I had never heard Lyndon call my name, or anyone's for that matter. He was smiling broadly, and his eyes were alive and animated. As he got closer, he grabbed me by my arm and hugged me. "Man, is it good to see you!" He looked around at the hallway. "It is great to be back here!"

"How are you, Lyndon?" I managed to squeak out, dumbstruck.

"Oh, I'm great now! Man, that place they took me to was AW-FUL! I can't even tell you! The food, the rooms—the nurses. I tell you, everything about that place was just the worst. I missed this place something awful. *Man, I'm glad to be home.*"

From that day forward, we witnessed a new Lyndon, and he never, as far as I could tell, went back to the old Lyndon again.

Lyndon's life story was punctuated by multiple layers and forms of injury: physical and emotional injury, received and inflicted. We never gained access to his origin story, mostly because no one knew how to ask. We don't know who he was before a newspaper clipping about a murder cast a dark ominous shade on him. Indeed, our relationship to criminality in our country asks that we not be attentive to the prequel, only the afterword. But having witnessed Lyndon's "reawakening," I would be remiss if I did not question the series of events, the societal forces, that precipitated the years of mental dormancy.

Jeanie, who had been victimized by Lyndon, never returned to The Space. Her family felt it was for the better: his change in countenance, after all, was no antidote to the brutal memory of his malignant footprint in her life; his changes had no power to clean up the carnage he'd left along the way.

There were other residents who had similarly troubling histories, but who were less menacing than Lyndon. The one I remember the most was named Vasquez. Vasquez was willing to spend extended periods talking about his history, despite its entanglements with gang life and gang-related activity. On one occasion, I visited Vasquez in the hospital, and he told me the story of his joining a gang, becoming infected, then getting out of the gang. As I sat by his bed he recounted that he came into his gang "through the back door," which meant he came in while in prison instead of on the streets. To hear Vasquez tell it, he did not need to come into the gang for protection—he didn't need protection from any street *hijos*—nor did he need a family. What he didn't have, what he was hungry for, was brothers (the fraternal type, had he been to college). And he was eager to find them in prison because that seemed to be where he was spending an inordinate amount of his time.

In fact, after a while, being locked up was all that he knew. He was first imprisoned at the age of fourteen. At that time, and in that detention center, it was mostly white kids—"they were backwoods *hermanos*; bad-backward-back-country-Klan-boys"—who wouldn't think anything of it to slice up the black and brown boys. Bad. So, the black and brown boys stuck together. This was when the Latin Kings took root in the predominantly white detention center: it was a matter of survival. "There were at least 500 of them and only about 180 of us blacks and Puerto Ricans, so even though we had different gangs, if you were black or brown you stuck together."

Vasquez spent the majority of his life—almost forty years—going through the revolving door of prison, then street life, then back to prison. "Always in the hole more than free." He remembered his early years in the gang fondly—the fast life, the women. Then one of the women he'd had a tryst with, a cream-colored Puerto Rican girl with brown hair and a cluster of freckles around her nose, started to get sick—very sick—and thin. There were whispers that she was dying, so, on a whim, he got an HIV test, and it came back positive.

That was when he said, *Si muero muero*—if I die, I die—because other than his gang, he had nothing to live for. Vasquez had been promoted to chief enforcer of his gang, and could anyone on the outside understand what that really meant? It meant if he told someone to stand and stare at a knife on the ground all day—just stand and stare at it—they did it. So, he maintained a sense of purpose, and tried to stay healthy, and continued to uphold his brotherhood with honor. And that was how he met Bea, the gang's bookkeeper, and a gem of a woman who kept such meticulous records that she could have worked for Ernst and Young, but for birth and circumstance.

But then the bust happened—DEA officers with guns drawn; dead presidents in flurries around them; a boot in Vasquez's back. The last thing he saw before the butt of a nine-millimeter hit him in the head was a Puerto Rican body falling across his back. There were the *policia blanquitos* with angry guns, and Bea crouching in the corner with a faint smile in the corner of her lips—then nothing.

Vasquez's right-hand man and his boss, the flunkies, the mules—even the little *amantes* who showed him a good time—all of them got twenty-five to life. Trafficking. Possession. Manufacturing. Dealing. (And worse.) Bea got twenty-five to life too, but having heard that Vasquez was dying, she'd removed his name from every record, and he walked. Every year since then, he sent Christmas and birthday gifts to Bea's daughter, a meager gesture of appreciation for saving his life.

When I met Vasquez he was down from a pack a day to three cigarettes a day, and the doctors considered him to be a model patient. When they told him to take his meds, he took his meds. When they said it was time for dialysis, he went to dialysis. When I went to visit him in the hospital, he offered me institutional tea in a styrofoam cup and we had rich conversations. When he had no visitors, he watched his soaps and did his crossword puzzle with his reading glasses propped on the tip of his nose. He didn't want much else, except to respect the people who enter his space, and have them respect him. "You know what I know, sis?" he said to me one day. "The rules in here are the same as the rules in jail, and in the gang, and in the drug game. The only difference is who's holding the needle."

That evening I left the hospital well after dark and walked to my car feeling the most incredible sensation of peace and understanding, deep understanding. The following week, Vasquez was readmitted to The Space from the hospital. As he thanked me for my visit the previous week I mentioned, "I hope I didn't seem rushed. My car was parked really far from the hospital, and it was really late." Vasquez looked at me and smiled.

"Remember the guy who came into the room and sat by you for a minute?"

I remembered him very well.

"I met him—and he became my brother—through Latin Kings," he said.

"Okay," I responded. He continued: "So between my room and your car, there wasn't nothing that could happen to you. Nothing."

Vasquez's stories captured the fanciful imaginings and the vague peril of gang life. After all, the persistence and popularity of mob and gangster narratives in American television, writing, and film encourage us to imagine that these life experiences are in another realm, that the violence and danger is confined to screens and pages. But Vasquez, in his storytelling, transformed the gang into a business—with bookkeepers and hierarchies, rules and deadlines. This normalizing of their daily obligations seemed to elevate his "career" from the underbelly of social norms to an above-ground "industry" that the government simply chose to criminalize. This reconstruction was profoundly validating for Vasquez.

Shortly after I met Vasquez, a fifty-year-old black man named Clyde moved in across the hall from Vasquez, and I started migrating to his room.

I learned very quickly that Clyde was a Vietnam vet and that he blamed the war, indirectly, for his diagnosis. He was only eighteen years old when he found out that he was being sent to Vietnam. The morning he got his orders, his mother looked at the papers, put them on the table, and locked herself in her room. It was only the three of them—Clyde, his mom, and his little brother.

One morning, a week before he was scheduled to leave, his mom made him breakfast—scrambled eggs—then sent him to wake up his little brother. He went into his brother's room and called to him, but his brother didn't answer. He knew, as soon as he turned him over, that his brother was dead. He stood there and stared at his brother for a long time.

His brother had had a heart attack, the result of a longstanding heart problem that the doctors at the local clinic said was probably minor. He went to get his mother, and for hours the two cried and cried, at the foot of the bed, across his body, outside the room, and holding his hand. Finally, they called for help.

The next week, just like Uncle Sam said, Clyde was off. He did not attend his brother's funeral.

They didn't know what they were doing over there. The only thing he recalls was shoot first or get shot. And he did get shot. Despite growing up in the housing projects of Chicago, the first time he saw a gun, picked it up, and fired it was in Vietnam. And the first person he shot was a small child—about seven or eight—who was pointing a gun at him. In a split second Clyde raised his gun and fired right at the child's head, and a woman he hadn't noticed before ran over to the child and threw herself over the child's body. At that moment he was transported back to Chicago and his mother laying across his dead brother's body. That was the moment he began to hate himself, and his spirit yearned for something to dim that image—a drug, a drink, a woman—anything.

Seventeen months in the trenches, moving like a trepid shadow, sleeping with his eyes open, waiting for death and hoping it would come with gentle swiftness. They ate when they could. Laughed when they could. Shat when they could. In a constant state of fear, with infections brewing in their feet, their genitals, their eyes, they learned that Vietnam was the incarnation of hell for any American man-child unfortunate enough to be stuck in its murderous clutches.

The Viet Cong eventually got him. He was in a trench when all of a sudden a sharp pain ripped through his back, then his leg. He turned and saw a Vietnamese soldier in a tree, his gun pointed directly at Clyde. As steadily as he could with his back and legs on fire, he shot the soldier clear out of the tree—or so he thought. Because the soldier had tied his leg to the tree, he fell backward, his gun hitting the floor. And as his body swung from the tree, his leg still securely fastened to a rope, Clyde found himself eye to eye with the enemy. Clyde was looking at him, but the other soldier was looking straight through Clyde. Clyde picked up the soldier's gun and shot him again.

That incident was Clyde's ticket home.

When he returned from Vietnam his country wasn't his anymore: like many vets, he was treated badly, as if he'd independently made the decision to fight a war. He was still a kid, not particularly invested in politics or policy. His government had sent him to fight a war that didn't benefit him, or his old neighborhood, or any ghetto for that matter. He didn't want special treatment because he was a vet. He just wanted not to be demonized after his country told him to be a killer, or get killed. Thankfully, most people ignored returning vets, but the folks who paid attention to them called them names that soldiers reserved for the Viet Cong.

He returned to his mother's house and everything was the same—except no money. He tried to get a job, but everything was under the table. Struggling during the day and being haunted by memories of war at night was too much. He took any small job he could get to help his mother make ends meet. With the income from the little jobs, he got some marijuana to help dull the pain. First he was using, then selling, then both.

He would get high to forget that nothing ever happens. He would get drunk to forget that a lot of things had happened. When life was bitterly cold, "the life" was warm and inviting. That was around the time he shot up for the first time. And that was probably how he contracted the virus.

When I met Clyde, he was five years clean. "I wake up and think about what I need to do today and I do it best I can. And I try to be decent to people. And that's it. It sounds crazy, but life has become something simple."

What struck me about Clyde's experience was that battle, after the war, became the persistent narrative of his life. Clyde fought in the war, then battled drugs, then the streets, then HIV/AIDS. His ability to talk about his experiences in the war became (he later recounted) an opportunity to move the stories "out of his head." This was liberating for Clyde.

Across the hall from Clyde was a woman named Nala whose room door was always closed. Every day Clyde would knock on her room door. When she shouted, "Come in," he would peek his head in hesitantly and say, "Just checking on you."

"Thank you, amigo," she would say. That would be the beginning and end of their interaction. Nala was a short, bulky Hispanic woman with cropped hair. She was in her mid-thirties, although she looked twenty-one. Nala had full-blown AIDS and a series of complications that resulted in a dim prognosis.

Nala had few visitors, which, generally speaking, was unusual for Hispanic residents, who seemed to be particularly successful at maintaining family ties that the disease seemed able to sever among most groups. The first day I went to see her was her birthday, so I ran out and bought her a pair of slippers and a painted wooden cross to hang on her wall. She thanked me for the gifts, noting "I thought my family and my *hijo* would come by. But they aren't coming." Nala had been clean for two months, but felt that few people had confidence that she could change behaviors that had persisted for twelve years. So her family didn't bother with her. The doctors told her that she had slow bleeding from the brain, and yet she felt she was getting stronger every day, and her memory, more and more acute. "I know that I am experiencing a miracle," she said. "I am going to live." But what was the point without her family and her son? Her girlfriend of two years had also absented herself. Even if she could get better, who would be waiting for her?

Her birthday came and went, and her momentary optimism turned into despair again. "I don't cry outside," Nala said, "but tears are rushing in my head, in my brain. Inside, my head is crying, crying, and I hold my head so the tears won't flood out." Three days later, Nala was dead. It was then, after her death, that the father of her son came to retrieve some items so the boy would remember his mother. I sat with him in her room for a while.

He met Nala at a Spanish prayer service in Bridgeport; she was twenty-four and he was fifty-two. People in the church community told him that she was a crack addict, and that she was homeless. He lived alone, and minded his business, and didn't run around with women. Although he only had a very small apartment, he was willing to take her in. So she went home with him. She made a bed on the floor and she was neat, and clean, and respected his place.

Weeks turned into months, and she was still there, always asking for money. At first he said no, but the longer she was there, the more he felt that he would rather give her money for drugs than think about her sticking up old ladies on the street, or selling herself. He never approached her sexually. He got up and went to work everyday, fixing anything people needed fixed in their homes. He didn't know what she did all day, but he suspected very little. So he gave her money. It wasn't long before she started to bring people to his house. Women. All kinds of women. He said to her, "Do what you want, but you can't be doing whatever with whoever in my house." After that she went out more and more—getting high, meeting up with all kinds of women, he heard.

One night she came home high and wanted to have sex with him. She'd never had sex with a man—in fact before she stayed with him she stayed as far away from men as possible. He felt confused, and resistant, and honored. He'd felt like a father-figure to her, so he said no. Instead, they snuggled, and then each night they started to snuggle, and the bed on the floor no longer served a purpose. Then one very cold night, it happened—one time—and four weeks later Nala told him she was pregnant.

He was going to be a father.

It's scandalous, people said. *She doesn't even LIKE men! And she runs the street all day.*

She stayed with him through her entire pregnancy, and after her period of intense morning sickness ended, she wanted to start going out again; she wanted to find more drugs.

"Absolutely NO!" he insisted, and he tried everything to stop her. But what could he do? She resumed her pleading for money, and threatened to get it from other people—by any means—if he wouldn't help her. *You're crazy*, people told him, *caring for a pregnant crack head—the worst kind of crack head there is.* But she was carrying his child, and the baby was now his responsibility, even if she wasn't.

Drugs provoked early labor. And he was sitting in the waiting room making a list of jobs he had over the next few days when a doctor came in and told him that the baby had to get medicine "because it had some kind of virus," he said.

"What kind of virus?" he asked.

"You don't know?" the doctor replied, then sighed. "Sir, I suggest you go in and ask the mother."

That's when she told him that she'd been HIV-positive for the past six years. The baby was beautiful when his face wasn't contorted and he wasn't shaking violently.

Through blinding anger, he went and got tested, and he was negative. On the baby's second day of life a social worker sat them down and told them that they had to take the baby for a full evaluation. He didn't know what that meant, or what it included. Worst of all, he didn't know what questions to ask. He signed the papers, and they left the hospital without the baby boy.

Days passed and he continually called the hospital to find out about the baby coming home, but message after message went unreturned. Finally, he went down to the hospital and found the nurse who had taken care of Nala. "Don't you know?" she asked. "You're not getting that baby back. They are taking custody away from you."

Unbelieving, utterly shocked and infuriated, he turned and ran, ran all the way home to tell Nala. But when he got home she was gone—gone to find drugs. Except this time was different. Her pillow was gone, and her knapsack, and her little Bible, and those were really the only things she had in this world. She was gone.

He went to a neighboring town where he knew there was a Puerto Rican lawyer who helped people with immigration issues. He didn't have an appointment, so he sat, and sat—the lawyer's secretary looking at him with bored indifference. When he finally got to see him he told him what happened, and that he wanted his baby. The lawyer told him to come back with $1500. So he went to the bank that same day, got the money, and went right back to the lawyer's office.

The lawyer looked at the money, and said, "Sir, why do you want this baby anyway? He's crack-addicted, and probably mentally handicapped and has AIDS."

Neither he, nor the lawyer, really knew the difference between HIV and AIDS. It didn't matter.

"I want him because he is mine," he said. He used his last savings in this world to get himself a suit and a haircut. In the end, the judge, hearing all of the evidence, turned to him solemnly and said, "Sir, what has happened to you—the way your son was taken away—was not fair. You are a good and decent man, and your son is a very lucky boy. You both will have a good life together. Return this man's son to him."

And that was exactly what happened. I met him eight years later. Eight years had gone by, and he was the father of a strong, beautiful boy who was HIV-negative. Nala came in and out of their lives for several years. Then, about a year before I met them, she disappeared. The next time someone mentioned Nala to him, it was to tell him that she was dying.

He took his son to see her once, but she didn't seem aware that they were there. He was also mindful not to stay long, for fear that his son would feel even a tingle of attachment. But, at the request of his son, they returned to her hospice room after her death so that the boy could find something to remember his mother. There wasn't much, so he took the cross from the wall.

"She lived how she wanted to live. In her way she loved me, and I loved her. And she give me my son. For that, I thank her."

Interestingly, the pairing of two versions of the same story from two different perspectives had the impact of reconstructing subjectivity for both parties. Rather than leaving the narratives triumphant (for him) and physically tragic (for her), together they present life stories that do not require approval or redemption. In the end both parties receive something more useful than a happy ending: they were liberated from the isolation of silence.

I know you are tired but come, this is the way.

—RUMI

4

Nine Deaths

She is a thorn, some say. *Just thorny*, others note. Slippery, tricky, kind, sweet, she doesn't deserve this. Complicated.

Why so much clamor?

The truth? She's a *child*.

Mariah was a small, wiry, biracial girl with large, yellow-ish eyes and shoulder-length, paper-thin brown hair covered, in patches, with a Crayola-box variety of colors. Although she was seventeen, no part of her appeared to have aged past eleven.

The first time I met Mariah, I was preparing to do a prayer service in the art room and several residents had already started to gather. After about seven residents found their way into the art room—by wheelchair, leaning on walkers, and upright on foot—I said, "Let's begin, friends, by asking God's presence with us today." I bowed my head, when suddenly the boom of hip-hop blared around us. I looked up and saw that the wiry girl, Mariah, had turned on the radio and—with full awareness that we were begin-ning a prayer service—stood before the group bobbing her head to the beat of the music, eyes closed, refusing to concede to the mood around her.

I stood up and walked over to the stereo. Reaching past her bobbing head, I turned the volume all the way down. I smiled. "We're beginning prayer service," I said. "We'd love for you to join us."

She looked at me blankly, shrugged her shoulders, and slouched down in a chair. I felt some nervousness, in part because I had never seen someone so young—so small—in residence at this facility. Moreover, who had put her here? Why was she sent to live in this facility, with all of these adults, seasoned through years—often decades—of street life? What had she done *already* to earn this fate? And what would be the key to her survival? My heart wanted to whisper, "I'm sorry . . . "

I sat down. The other residents looked at me, as if they needed me to make sense of the new girl. By the time I finished our opening prayer and looked back in her direction, she was fast asleep, snoring loudly, with her head hanging back and her mouth wide open, bearing a mouthful of haphazardly arranged and double-rowed teeth. When I suggested, next, that we sing, she was shaken awake by our clapping, and after taking a second to reorient herself to her surroundings, she wiped some drool from her mouth, sucked her teeth, and walked out of the art room lazily, and without looking back.

I waited a few days before going to see her.

Mariah was born with the virus. Her father was a black drug dealer, her mother a white drug addict. Mariah's mother turned her over to be raised by her black grandparents shortly after both she and Mariah's father were diagnosed with the virus. She never knew her father. Her mother proceeded to come in and out of her life—often hitting Mariah's grandparents up for money. Mariah spent her early life in good health; in fact, neither her school nor her school classmates knew she had the virus. Their home, however, was painfully chaotic and oftentimes unlivable. It housed a gaggle of brothers (her mother's other children from various relationships) and cousins—all male—and she never had her own room. Her entire life, she'd fashioned a living room couch into a bed and bedroom. It was never clear where all of these boys slept, but no one doubted that the presence of so many males of varying ages left Mariah open to abuse. Mariah's grandmother, her primary caregiver, was an obese and evangelically religious woman. She could barely walk, but what she lacked in mobility she made up for in audibility, loquaciously sharing thoughts that ran the gamut from praise to condemnation. She thought Mariah didn't need pain medicine, because suffering was an important test of faith. She believed that Mariah sabotaged God's desire to heal her because of her lack of faith. She prayed loudly and argued loudly and talked about reality shows vigorously. She was, if nothing else, consistent.

Mariah did not care for school. She made some friends, but none of them ever became close enough that she shared her diagnosis or discussed her chaotic home situation. When she became a teenager, she didn't tell the boys she slept with. In fact, at one point it was rumored that she had come to The Space to hide from a former boyfriend who tested positive and was looking for her.

When Mariah did go to school, she found her way to a rough crowd, and was in and out of trouble. She was suspended from school often, usually for fighting, a hard thing to imagine when looking at her unusually tiny frame.

At the age of fourteen, she started getting symptoms. By fifteen, she dealt with bouts of PCP and thrush—in addition to a huge cyst covering part of her face and ear—and low blood counts. She looked as desperately ill as she was.

The first time I visited her in her room, I started by explaining to her what a chaplain is.

"How old are you?" I asked her.

"Seventeen. How old are you?"

I looked at her for a moment, startled. "Thirty-three," I responded.

"Dang! You don't look that old! You look like … like … I don't know, but not old like that!"

"That's good," I smiled at her. "So, do you want to talk about how you came to be here?"

She looked into space then shrugged her shoulders absently, "I dunno." She picked at a scab on her elbow. "Why would you want to work here anyway? You couldn't find another job?"

"I like it here. I like meeting different people. Helping people when I can."

"Umph. This place? This place is depressing. I wouldn't be here if I didn't have to. Your parents alive?"

"They're alive."

We went on like this—playing twenty questions with each other—for over an hour.

Mariah's biggest problem at The Space was the thing that made her case so tragic: her age. Older residents—male and female—would attempt to prey on her in various ways. Many wanted to be her friend because she was young and pretty. Many sought her out because they thought she was naïve. Some befriended her because they thought the staff was more empathetic towards her, and tried to affix themselves to her good favor.

But the truth was that, among the staff, Mariah would fall in and out of favor on a daily basis. There were nurses and nurses' aides who regularly brought her treats, like McDonald's and KFC. Such behaviors would anger the dietician, who accused the offending staffers of sabotaging Mariah's well-being. Mariah, on the other hand, was savvy enough to work a room, and to calculate where and with whom to build an alliance on any given day.

Mariah often claimed she was too sick to come to the dining room, and demanded dinner in bed. When she did come to the dining room, it was more often than not in her pajamas. One evening, after the day staff had clocked out, Mariah begrudgingly made her way to the dining room for dinner. A few minutes after receiving her plated dinner, she began to complain loudly that her chicken was not cooked. She proceeded to rally other residents to refuse the chicken, tearing the skin back and exposing what she claimed was bright pink flesh. After pushing her tray away, she retreated to her room. The next day, the Board of Health received an anonymous complaint. Most of the kitchen staff felt certain that the call was made by Mariah, and, in Mariah's opinion, she was "blacklisted" by the kitchen staff.

Mariah started refusing to take her meals in the dining room. When the tray was brought to her room, she would often refuse to eat there too, commenting to me that "these people are nasty." Sometimes she would proclaim more animatedly that "white people are nasty," showing no partiality to her own pale skin and straight hair.

I was not a part of the solution: I brought food for Mariah—usually a Big Mac and a milkshake—on more than one occasion, in response to her daily wide-eyed plea "Do you think you could bring me just one thing from McDonald's?"

I always asked our dietician before bringing Mariah treats, and she would usually tell me what I already knew: an endless assortment of "treats" was not the answer. Yes, Mariah was young, and paper thin, and probably hungry *for what she wanted*. But she was also a resident at a facility where residents ate what was given to them in the interest of their health. She was the "pet" of too many staffers. It was alarming how often members of the maintenance staff sat in her room—mops still in hand—watching Jerry Springer and reality shows with her. Mariah even told me that one staff member, on the way back from a doctor's appointment, took Mariah to her house to meet her dogs.

Mariah knew when to plead innocence and when to play tough. She knew when to be sweet and when to play hardball. But she suffered from authentic, unaffected arrested development. And when she would ask me an endless string of questions, she wanted—in a sophomoric and innocent way—to know the real answers. She was demonstrating the wide-eyed, unfiltered curiosity of a normal young child. She was savvy and naïve, culpable yet above suspicion.

Over the course of the next two years I spent countless hours with her, often sitting on her bed, talking about living and dying, and brushing Mariah's hair. Getting her hair brushed and braided—often in two or four ponytails, like a six-year-old girl—was her favorite thing. She lived in a great deal of pain much of the time, and she had chronic insomnia; but having her hair brushed was one thing that lulled her to sleep without fail. We would usually begin our time together by getting caught up on the facility's goings on: Who was in trouble, and for what offense? Then I would ask her about her specific prayer requests for the day. Having been raised by evangelicals, her belief in God was rooted in muscle memory, and she quickly regurgitated phrases like "He needs Jesus!" and "Someone needs to pray for that girl." She always held my hands during prayer. She held them so tightly it felt like she was clinging to conviction, after which she would lie down, and I would brush her hair until she fell asleep.

Mariah came and left The Space half a dozen times in the four and a half years I knew her. Sometimes she would be put on restriction for violating rules. She was caught smoking in her room on several occasions, and at other times she refused medication in dramatic tantrums, which caused her to be "charged" with being medically noncompliant. Once she was placed on restriction she would pack her things in a half dozen garbage bags and have a relative pick her up. A few weeks later she would be back with the same bags.

Mariah tended to befriend the less popular residents, and would often be seen having a cigarette with a resident named Marlon, who floated along the margins and was often ridiculed for his slow meandering speech, except when Mariah was around. She could also be found with Parks, who, despite his heavy-set, heavy-handed demeanor with most of us, softened and surrendered his bulldoggish posture when having a cigarette with Mariah.

The first time Mariah returned to us with full-blown AIDS, she had shrunk from her usually thin self to a skeletal frame. Her cheeks were sunken and her skin was jaundiced. Her hair had started to fall out, and her arms had broken out in sores that were wrapped in two heavy casts of gauze. She still wanted to have her hair brushed, but when her hair started coming out in patches, I took to massaging her scalp instead. Mariah was afraid of dying. She was afraid that death was a dark and lonely place. During one of our many conversations about death I shared with her my belief that death was complete light, and clarity, and peace. Death looked and smelled and felt like springtime—a luminous, beaming rebirth. For fleeting moments, she seemed to believe me.

For fleeting moments, I believed myself.

When Mariah left the next time, it was because her family announced that they were moving to North Carolina. At the time that she told us this, they hadn't yet secured a place to live. Also, it wasn't clear who—of the many people living in their home—had been invited to go. But I began to hear whisperings that taking Mariah to North Carolina had never been a part of the family's plan, and—in fact—they had not made any medical provisions for her relocation.

From what the staff could gather, the family was going to North Carolina, but she was staying with us.

After several cycles of going home, coming back to The Space, and going home again, Mariah's condition continued to deteriorate. When she was moved from The Space to the hospital, her request remained the same: to have her hair brushed. I continued braiding her now wispy hair in two or four ponytails, with rubber bands binding them. She would leave the little girl plaits in until I offered to comb her hair again.

One day, after returning from the hospital, Mariah, rail-thin and pale, volunteered to sing at a prayer service at The Space. A steady soulful voice filled the room, and the nurses paused at their station.

The residents abandoned their bickering, snoozing, and gossiping—and the staff stopped too. The maintenance workers stopped, mops and dust rags in hand. A member of the kitchen staff, who had been straightening up the coffee station, paused deliberately. The more I watched Mariah, the more I observed her— her frame, her delicate facial features—the more I was completely overwhelmed with joy and grief.

The fifth time Mariah returned to us, I was forewarned that she'd decided to hole up in her room. She was in more pain than I'd ever seen her in, constant and unrelenting pain all over her body. When I walked into her room the blinds were shut (the light bothered her eyes) and she was curled up in the middle of the bed crying. I shut off the bellowing, scandalous television program she had on and found her hairbrush. I brushed her hair and hummed softly. Little by little her sobs turned to whimpers, until she fell asleep. Within a week, she asked to go home, went, was sent back to us, then admitted to the hospital.

"How are you?" I asked, when I called her at the hospital.

"Terrible," she said, in a dispirited whisper. "This sucks. When are you coming to see me?"

"Soon," I told her.

"Good," she said, hardly audible. "I'm bored."

The next day Mariah died.

I drove an hour to her funeral, only to discover that her family had canceled the service. We were never told when or where she was buried.

Because she was ill for most of her life, Mariah may not have fully established a counter-discourse to illness that allowed her to put her suffering in perspective. The social construction of her body, and its sense of belonging in the world, was dependent upon doctors and nurses, and an overcrowded and under-attentive home. Her questions made sense: they were a way for her to gather information and to engage others in the normal developmental process that allows us to see ourselves as interactive agents rather than victims.

Mariah had one real friend during her time at The Space: a misanthrope named Parks. Parks was a heavy-set fifty-something black man whose arms were always defensively strapped across his massive wheelchair-bound frame in what appeared to me to be an unprovoked state of defiance. He struggled with profound ambivalence about his existence, his purpose, and even his own ability to develop relationships with those around him. He was disinterested in those who, like him, were infected, and he was hostile towards those of us who weren't. To say that the word "friend" crept into my relationship with Parks slowly and unexpectedly is to say little to nothing of the strange relationship that evolved between us. Parks was, by any measure, a disagreeable misanthrope. His mouth was fixed in a permanent pout, and he bore an unrelenting furrow in his eyebrows. Even when he laughed (and he did not laugh frequently or easily) his eyes continued to frown. His posture towards those around him vacillated between a slump of hopelessness and obvious irritation—unless he was flat out ignoring you, in which case he would deny your existence altogether.

The first time I approached him he looked up from his color-by-number painting, glanced at me, briefly, then continued coloring. "What do *you* want?"

"I just wanted to say hello," I responded, feeling like the nerd inching toward the cool kids' lunch table.

"So?" he asked.

"So, I just wanted to say hello," I repeated, with equal trepidation.

"Good. Done. Bye." Parks said, coloring more vigorously.

Parks interacted with me this way for months, when he interacted with me at all. Sometimes he'd render me invisible. On days when I ignored him he would respond in the opposite manner, yelling insults at me across the room: "Call yourself a spiritual person? You see anyone gettin' religion 'round here? You a joke." Other times he'd bark orders at me: "You got nothing but time— why don't you go get me a bag of chips. The next day he said, "You back here again? Ain't you had enough yet?"

"I'm back," I said plainly. "Why wouldn't I be?"

"Then you must love punishment. Or maybe you just a plain fool, 'cause most people come a while then don't nobody see them no more. You must just love punishment is all."

"Mind if I sit and paint with you?" I asked.

"I ain't your mammy. Do whatever you want."

Thus went our relationship for the next two years, with a few occasions when I "gave up" on him, and many, I imagine, when he gave up on me. On Parks's birthday, I brought him—with his nurse's permission—a "treat" of his favorite food: Kentucky Fried Chicken hot wings and potato wedges.

"Who ever heard of giving wings as a birthday gift?" he complained. "This all you brought me?" A week before Christmas I brought Parks an extra, extra large and very warm Georgetown sweatshirt, the gift he'd requested for Christmas as part of our annual staff-resident "Secret Santa." "This is too small ..." he barked, holding it up like a dust rag. "Looks like I wind up with what I usually get—nothing. . . ."

He also told me that as long as I'd been seeing him I must have known, clear as day, that that size would not fit him, so I must have given the sweatshirt to him with the thought of taking it back in the first place.

I decided that day that I was fed up with Parks, and I told him that he could do what he wanted with the sweatshirt, and I hoped he had a peaceful Christmas. Later that week I saw a nurse's aide wearing the sweatshirt.

During the summer of that same year I went on a vacation and when I returned, Parks's eyes latched onto me as I chatted with nurses and other staff. Suddenly he yelled out, "Nice of you to come back. You've been gone eight days."

I smiled. This was my first victory. I was moved that he'd been counting the days, but, more so, I was struck by how long the days must seem when you are well of mind and sick of body, spending many hours, like Parks, painting pictures, dawdling the hours between meals, and hoping for visitors.

"How are you doing?" I asked, ready for the weekly reprimand.

"Huh, I'll tell you how I am doing. Terrible. Just like you see me, that's just how I am. And if you want to do something for me you can get me out of this place. Or save yourself and get out of here, which is what everyone does eventually anyway."

My way of dealing with Parks here forward was humor. First, I would tell him about the getaway car out front, then I would tease him about his grumpiness, and eventually I would rub his head and make light of his funny hair, which was short, soft, and determined to grow in many different directions. "Has your hair figured out which way to go?" I would tease. "Go away," he would respond with a half smile.

One day he added: "you don't come 'round here enough." That was the closest thing to a compliment I ever got from Parks.

On that day he was lying on his side with his legs hanging over the bed. Both of his ankles were severely swollen, fully bandaged, and bleeding through the bandages. His feet, blackened and bubbling, looked as though they had survived a fire. His eyes were downcast, staring with great intensity at a small pool of blood on the floor.

"I hate myself," he said.

"You hate your illness?" I asked.

He shook his head, "All of it. All of it. Look at me! I'm disgusting. I'm always in pain. I hate this life. I don't want to be here anymore. The ones who die are the lucky ones. I just want to die."

I leaned close to him and held his hand.

He began to shake his head and mumble. Among his mumbles he repeated over and over that he wanted to be in the hospital.

"Nobody cares." He tried to lean back and couldn't, because of an intense shooting pain in his back. He tried to lean forward and couldn't, because of cramping in his stomach. His frustration escalated.

"I care," I said, and tightened my grip on his hand. Tears began to roll down his cheeks. I dried his eyes with a napkin. As I ran out of words, I focused on catching his tears as they fell.

"Tell me about a time when you liked being alive," I said. He hesitated, then talked in a labored voice, and through his own tears, about a better time. "I was a mischievous kid, I guess. Bad. Just like now. A problem to everyone. But I took care of my mother. I always worked and took care of my mother."

"Is she still living?" I asked, and he responded that she wasn't.

He went on to tell me that he spent his childhood working, when and where he could, to give money to his mother and to help take care of his sister. As he got older, he turned to drinking to help deal with stress in his life. It was while drunk, he believes, that he had unprotected sex and contracted the virus. Before his diagnosis, there had been many years of feeling overworked, low on energy, and lethargic. He had only found out about his AIDS diagnosis one month before I met him.

The risk that Parks took in speaking through any emotion other than anger prompted me to exercise some reciprocal vulnerability. I sat next to him on his bed and we held hands. After a while I spoke: "If I walked into this place tomorrow and you were not here, my life would not be the same. Your life matters a great deal to me."

I waited for the insults, but instead Parks let go and wept like a small baby. He wept and wept and wept.

I continued to visit Parks over the next few months. In between his sarcastic comments and dismissive utterances, he told me about his dream of getting his own apartment and making a life for himself on the "outside."

During one such conversation he mentioned that his doctor wanted to send him to the hospital. He had an infection that wouldn't go away and was getting worse. Over the next few weeks, the infection spread from a sore on his ankle, to patches traveling up his massive legs. One day he went to bed and slept all day, then all of the next day. During this second day of sleep a nurse went to bring him his dinner and found him minimally responsive. It was discovered that he had had a stroke. He was moved to the hospital where he went in and out of slumber. Before work, after leaving The Space, on my way to do grocery shopping—one way or another—I visited him everyday.

He became, over the course of the next few weeks, a ritual in my life, like brushing my teeth, like shutting off the alarm clock, like knowing how to drive. I spent hours talking with him as he drifted in and out of slumber. I read the newspaper to him. I sang to him too, until he demanded, with arrested breath, that I "cut it out." When he finally slipped into a coma, I made a bed out of two chairs in his hospital room and stayed with him until late in the evening. I didn't care about healthy boundaries, or chaplaincy being driven by prayerfulness, or patient-client social contracts. He'd become my friend, which said everything about my breaching of professional frontiers and nothing of balancing his needs and my spiritual practices as separate entities.

I questioned, for the first time, if my caregiving was healthy, or anywhere near normal. Being a chaplain was my job, and he was my client. When I "punched out" at The Space and then spent hours with dying residents, I, without fully realizing it at the time, was asking them to fill a need of mine, but what was it? Maybe my giving—maybe all giving—was privately selfish, self-congratulatory. Maybe there was a piece of me that used the suffering of others to feel useful in my own small, inconsequential life. Or—most terrifying of all—perhaps I needed people to pass so that I could have closure for myself. I was not so much sitting with them through their death process as I was *waiting out* their death process. *Is waiting for death*, I started to wonder, *the same as caring for a life?* Bedside death rituals are meant for families, I told myself, not care workers who must move forward to tend to the next fragile bedside.

I decided to cut back on my time with Parks; at the very least, I stopped making a bed out of chairs in his room and lying there for hours dozing, with the television fading in and out. I was two days into questioning my leaking emotional margins when I received a call telling me that Parks had died.

Eulogizing Parks at the small memorial service his family planned for him was one of the most important occasions of my time in ministry. First, because of the obvious: I had grown to love him; but also, because everyone from his family to his caregivers had felt challenged in finding a way to love him, given his abrasive exterior.

I needed Parks's eulogy to speak to the worthiness of questioning difficult journeys and to give legitimacy to our temporal displeasure with God. Were Parks a prophet he couldn't have spoken more acutely to the plight of the suffering servant. But even in the midst of Parks's suffering—in his dissatisfaction with unanswered questions—he did, indeed, *live*. Even when Parks was disgruntled, he made art, works that bore witness to his desire for beauty, and tranquility, and peace. He had a quick wit, and clear eyes, and he knew when to push people and when to back off.

Parks's death was one of many I had to "bear witness" to, both for the deceased and for those who were called to survive. One of my responsibilities as chaplain was to talk to residents about their impending deaths. It's a disquieting job, and naturally, more of a conversation about wishes than a statement about mortality. It hadn't occurred to me prior to taking this position that I would be asked so often to discuss death as a "life occasion." Contrary to what I previously thought (or hadn't thought about), we don't instinctually know we are dying, and, that said, we have a right to know. Moreover, when our curiosity about mortality is well-fed, we have more opportunities to feel a peace both inward- and outward-facing.

A resident named Marlon, who befriended Mariah and Parks, made a special request to attend Parks's funeral service, which was forty miles away. Actually, he attended every funeral service, prayer service, religious holiday service, and Bible study. If there was an occasion to offer a prayer petition, Marlon always spoke up.

"I want to pray for better food. Because the food here is killing me," he would say, in his sleepy southern drawl.

"Well, the Lord is certainly concerned about *all* of our troubles," I would often tell him. "And while we can ask Him anything—really, anything!—we can also give thanks for what we have right now."

"But I want fried chicken. And greens."

On this particular occasion, a resident in the corner got antsy in his wheelchair. "Awright-already, fried chicken, Amen, move on."

"I'm just sayin' . . ." Marlon continues.

"It's the same thing every week," another resident barks at Marlon, "fried chicken, fried chicken. Fried friggin' chicken. What *is* it with you and the fried chicken?"

Marlon thought about it. I opened my mouth to move on but waited, because Marlon seemed to be preparing to answer the question. "Well, last week we did have fried chicken. And rice. And mixed vegetables. Only eat the carrots though. And pudding . . .

but that night—*that* night—the chicken was all pink-like inside. So I figure that that night don't count."

Through it all, a resident sat staring at me, pleading with her eyes that I stop the chicken talk.

The laundry list of concerns never got shorter, and whether they were of the mercurial sort or grave, Marlon asked that his prayer requests be welcomed with equal energy.

One day, my supervisor informed me that a resident named Omez, who had been taken to the hospital, was dying. After leaving The Space I went to spend time with him. By the time I arrived at the hospital he had slipped into a coma. A minister was at his bedside along with a woman who had been assigned by the hospital as his case worker.

Omez's nurse informed me that I was just in time, because they were preparing to extubate him. As we waited for the attending physician, we—the hospital minister, the case worker, and I—talked quietly about nothing in particular, and before long the attending physician, a small man with exceptionally gentle eyes, informed us that Omez would probably survive only a few minutes after his tubes had been removed. As the minister and social worker tried to make small talk, I found myself leaking tears, then crying heavily. I was overcome with embarrassment over my inability to control myself. I'd been at the Space for a while now, but I'd never been present at the very moment life ended. The social worker patted my back, wondering, I imagine, how a chaplain could be such a mess.

"It's good that you are here as Omez is transitioning. It's okay," she said to me.

"I didn't know he was dying when I came," I said, almost as a confession. "I've never seen … this is the first time I've been present . . . ."

What a fruitless, meaningless confession, I thought.

At that moment, the doctor came out and told us that we could go in. The social worker nudged me forward.

I felt Omez's warm and shallow breaths, and the utter peacefulness of his expression. The beeping of unsympathetic machines sounded a somber symphony around us.

"Omez was lucky to have so many people caring for him. He was a very lucky man, indeed." the nurse said.

It seemed to be meaningless chatter. What's lucky about being thirty-four years old, lying on your death bed after ten years of being in and out of crack houses, and not a single family member to sit by your bedside—or bury you?

Then the beeps—the symphony—became a steady streaming tone, which was hurriedly shut off by the doctor. And the whole time, my hand was on Omez's forehead. There was a natural pause in the conversation, and the doctor glanced at his watch through respectfully crossed hands to say, "Omez is gone. He didn't suffer. He did not suffer at all."

And at that moment, I looked at Omez, and I pressed my hand firmly against his head. My grief dissipated. I thought, *Make haste; this world had nothing more to give you*. And at that instant the tears dried from my cheeks and the sadness and pain were extracted from my spirit—fleeing from my body. My hand was still on Omez when I began to feel a peace come over me, almost as if I was being gifted a piece of his release—a piece of his peace.

After leaving the hospital, I stepped into the New England night and I let my lungs fill with cold air. Cold, clear air. I walked, strong focused steps. Then I stopped and looked around. Suddenly I saw what looked like billions of disassembled pieces of sky, and streams of air floating around me, all—like a puzzle—being reassembled into matter. As I crossed the street and the streetlight changed, the sound of honking horns seemed to be blowing in harmony.

Omez. From his birth in a small shanty in Puerto Rico and mine in a city hospital in the Bronx, we came to a mutual time and place and I prayed with him and for him and wound up at his bedside, and something, in turn, some piece of his spirit—it felt—had been imparted to me. For a moment, I felt the most perfect freedom. In the middle of the street, with the honking harmony, I thought I was experiencing Nirvana.

Almost a week after Omez passed, Marlon died without getting his final serving of fried chicken. I planned a memorial service in their honor. The evening of the service I made several announcements inviting residents to join us in the prayer room at The Space to remember their friends.

At the designated time for the service I made my way to the prayer room and waited for others to arrive. Ten minutes later, a single resident rolled her wheelchair into the prayer room, after which she stretched out her legs, folded her arms, and drifted into a deep sleep.

With one person present, I began, "We have gathered here to remember our friends Marlon and Omez." The sleeping patient raised her body up slightly, then dropped her head heavily, and let out a thunderous snore.

I put down my Bible and the folded stack of colored paper. I sat in silence, staring at the sleeping lady. She looked peaceful. There we were, two gathered for two. I put my face in my hands and sighed heavily for the unremembered.

The sleeping mourner with the memorable snore was a fifty-year-old Hispanic woman named Ana. She had come here to die, but she wouldn't, and we all knew it. She arrived with full-blown AIDS, cancer throughout her entire upper body, and PCP (AIDS-related pneumonia). Ana was a paper-thin, olive-skinned woman with thick curly hair, keen sharp features, and disproportionately large and expressive brown eyes. Ana was a big hugger and kisser, and physical contact seemed to recharge her so fully that it seemed life was being injected into her based on how much affection she received each day. Because of throat cancer, she spoke in a raspy voice and she used her hands to substitute for the enthusiasm that her voice lacked.

I spent a good deal of time with Ana in prayer, and in conversation. One day, a doctor announced to us that Ana's organs were failing rapidly, and that she might not make it through the night. A death vigil orchestrated by nurses began by her bedside as she slept and woke. Her chest rattled and hummed. She moaned softly from time to time, and tears rolled intermittently from her eyes, proof, we thought, that her mind was still dreaming. Every now and then she would awake and ball her hands into resolute fists.

"It's okay, Ana," I said stroking her arm. "You're okay." I read to her from her Bible. She would settle down and begin her cycle again.

As each doctor, nurse, and fellow patient left her room, they offered solemn goodbyes. I left that day expecting to receive word of Ana's death the way I always received such information—the startling ring of my phone in the middle of the night.

But Ana did not die that day or that night. She didn't die the day after that or the day after that. Or even the day after *that*.

In fact, one month after Ana arrived at the Space, I came in to find Ana's rail-thin legs strolling awkwardly down the hallway in sweats and sneakers, her hair pulled up in a tidy scrunchy. She was wheezing greetings to nurses and doctors, waving cheerily and looking for hugs.

It was three months later—six hours after her youngest son arrived from Florida to visit—that Ana died.

Ana had told many of us that her son was coming to visit, but because he had promised to visit several times, and had failed to keep any promises, we did not encourage her hopefulness. Ana turned her back on death to wait for her youngest son.

I did not go to the prayer room to mourn for Ana after her death. In fact, I did not sit still for the next week. I moved to a new apartment; I witnessed the eleventh of September in 2001. I visited my father, who was in a hospital in New York undergoing cancer treatment.

Then in December, three hours before the New Year, I stopped. I took a deep breath and, upon exhaling, I cried for a long, long time. I cried for the tens of millions of people who had lost their lives because of AIDS-related illness since the disease's origin. I cried for the bodies scattered about lower Manhattan. I cried because too many people suffered.

About one hour after I started to cry, I took another long, deep breath and stopped.

I poked my swollen eyes and decided not to cry anymore.

The greatest difficulty that people living with HIV/AIDS face in a residential facility is watching other people suffer, while imagining what their own future holds. This was made especially clear to me after the death of one forty-six-year-old man named Leonard who had been with us for only two months before he died. After Leonard's death, the gentleman in the room next to him, named Devon, rolled his wheelchair through the front door of the facility without telling anyone, and did not return for several weeks. When he finally did return, he was given warning that if he left against medical advice again, he would not be permitted to return. When I went to talk to him, he slumped in his wheelchair, looking forlorn and depressed.

"When I heard that Leonard died, I took off out of here," he said. He rolled his wheelchair up the street, then up the next street, then up the street after that. He wasn't concerned with consequences or repercussions.

Devon shifted uncomfortably, as if he was contemplating whether it was worth it to talk to me or not. Then, with a sigh of surrender, he said, "When I was twelve my father was shot."

Devon was hanging out on a corner when someone came running up to tell him that his father had been shot right in front of their apartment. His father was doing drugs on other people's dime; he owed a lot of money. There were always rumors that people were looking for him. Devon took off around the corner and saw his father lying in the doorway of their building with blood all over him. He got down on his hands and knees and ordered his father not to die. "That's alright son," his father said, "my time here is up." And, just like that, his father was gone.

The local undertaker—his name was Mr. Oscar—came after what felt like an eternity and took his father's body away.

After that, Devon got into everything his parents had warned him about: he started selling drugs, then buying drugs. Once he crossed over and attempted to sell drugs on someone else's turf. Six burly guys he'd never seen before came looking for him, but by that point he didn't care anymore: he was no longer afraid—of anything. Devon just started swinging, and swinging, and while he doesn't remember passing out, he does remember that he didn't stop swinging. His hands bore witness to his years of fighting.

Eventually the law caught up with him, and he was prosecuted and sent to prison for drug possession and trafficking. And that was when he learned one of his most valuable life lessons: prison doesn't make people crazy; the absence of the elements of freedom—birds, air, trees, and touch—cause you to lose your mind.

Almost as if she had been waiting for him, Devon's mother died as soon as he was released, in the same apartment building where his father had died. And the very same man who had come to get his father twenty years earlier—Mr. Oscar— retrieved his mother's body. Devon cared about very little before his mother's death. Now he cared about nothing.

Devon spent the next few years in and out of jail. His exposure to death seemed to be marked by resounding silences—the undertaker who, on both occasions, had no words of comfort; his deceased parents whose deaths left silent spaces; the (presumably) invisible community, which faded into the distant background as Devon dealt with these traumas utterly alone.

Then one day, something happened that changed Devon even more dramatically, and irreparably. His girlfriend was sitting waiting for him in a car. Some men who had been looking for him saw his car and started shooting. And shooting. When they retreated, she was dead. It was shortly after that that Devon— already done with life— found out he was HIV-positive. He had been sick for a long time, mostly flu-ish, and without an appetite. Then, about a year after his diagnosis, he woke up unable to move his legs. He was taken to the hospital where a host of doctors used words like "opportunistic infection" and "ascending paralysis."

In addition to the silences that are left with the deaths of multiple loved ones—and in addition to the questions left unanswered within the silences—the woman he believed caused his infection never acknowledged it to him. She never provided an explanation, or apology, or clarification.

So when Leonard, whom Devon had known in the old neighborhood, came to The Space, he was surprised but happy to see him—and even happier that their rooms were side by side. The two were never close, but they knew each other's mothers, and each brought back better (or alternative) memories of the old neighborhood. But within a few days, Leonard had declined so dramatically that they couldn't carry on conversations. Then Devon saw family members, many of whom he remembered, coming out of Leonard's room crying. He just sat and watched outside the room door. And who should show up to retrieve Leonard's body? Mr. Oscar, smiling at him as if he was the twelve-year-old boy again. That was when Devon decided it was time to go.

"So I just took off. I felt like I needed to be free, and breathe fresh air. I went up the block, and up the next one. And the next one. I went eight whole blocks, and there I was in my old neighborhood. And I was in my wheelchair and I looked around, and do you know I saw them same guys—the same addicts—who were strung out on the street back in the day, still hanging around strung out on the same corners."

Devon stopped running long enough to think about the difficult questions. Why did these people, so loved, so essential to his existence, leave him? At whom will the undertaker smile next?

According to Elisabeth Kubler-Ross, we all share a basic belief that death is not part of what we think of as the experience of living—more strongly stated, "death is never possible in regard to *ourselves*," Kubler-Ross says—therefore, we all, on some level, attribute dying to some "malicious intervention from the outside by someone else." Death is subconsciously rationalized as a form of punishment.[1] This reaction to death, which is held on some level by all societies, explains why, when we witness the deaths of others, we reflexively question our own worthiness to live.

The most memorable relationship that I shared with a resident while at The Space was with a man named Law. When I met Law he was an old man, though he was relatively young in years—only sixty. Having spent most of his adult life in prison, he determined that he would spend what was left with books, and bird-watching, and viewing Audrey Hepburn movie marathons. My connection

1. Kubler-Ross, *On Death and Dying*, 2.

with Law was instant and organic, like an uncle I'd grown up with, like a college mentor, like the neighbor down the street who listens to you when your parents don't. Law liked to listen—he would thoughtfully look you squarely in the eyes, a finger poised on his cheek, as if he was processing the words as they left your lips.

During one of our innumerable conversations, Law recounted a dream he had of me in my role as chaplain at The Space. In his dream, he told me, I was surrounded by many people who loved me, but none of them could see my face. I was just skin—no eyes, no nose, no mouth. "This work you have taken on," he said slowly, "requires reciprocity. You give, we give. We suffer, you suffer. It's a yin-yang. Don't do it crooked." I thanked him for this insight, and promised to think about it. I got up to leave and he added, "By the way, all this time we've been talking I never asked you: You got kids?" I told him I didn't. "You need kids. Couple of girls. You're going to be a great mom."

"I'm not married yet," I laughed.

He picked up a plastic knife and started carving an apple. "Didn't say you needed a husband. Said you needed kids."

It seemed that God provided Law with insight that we all needed, including other residents, their family members, and staff. Five years later he was proven right about me. I did need children. And I didn't need a husband.

So Law was our resident prophet, the "Godfather," the go-to guy. In prison, he had also been highly regarded for his quiet wisdom and introspection. He read voraciously, and had a mental certainty that distinguished him from the masses. In the end, he had some sort of spiritual authority, an understood distinctiveness, and the staff granted him an existential version of tenure.

Six months after he told me to have children, Law died.

That was when an unexplainable series of events, with no precedent, visited The Space.

Law took with him every drop of peace at The Space, and left us in a circle of chaos that he himself—all by himself—orchestrated, then cultivated and pruned into full bloom. All those years, he had stood at the nexus of the staff and the residents, and without him our collective equilibrium was disrupted. Nurses seemed more impatient with each other and social workers less responsive. Nurses' aides were generally the toughest of all, solid rocks when the rest of us were weak. But now their strength morphed into coldness, indifference. Volunteers came less frequently, or so it seemed. A new patient didn't occupy Law's room for a long time, and we thought it was because it needed to be cleaned out, but there was nothing to clean after his family—whom none of us had seen, or met, or even heard of in the seven years he'd been with us—swooped in like falcons and took everything, including a yellowed, two-year-old wall calendar; including a worn leather shoe with no mate.

At lunch time, the usual whiff of fish and chips and warm chocolate chip cookies was gone, and the residents—gathering at nine, noon, and six for meals—ate in silence with downcast eyes.

Law *was* at the center of *all* of this. He had died very slowly, and it felt as if so much emotional attention had been focused on him for so long that our high regard for him—our child-like devotion—superseded our desire to act in the best interest of the whole. The medical staff might say it was the uniqueness of his case, and the nurses' aides might point out that his room was coincidentally closest to the nurses' station. Everyone had a reason for the ever-increasing significance of Law.

The truth is that Law had been so well-intentioned, but unsuccessful, in making peace with his mistakes, in exorcizing the ghosts of his past, that to create a clear passage for him out of this life we all, every one of us, had accepted his anger, his frustration, his paranoia—the film of his life that played over and over in his head, just behind the quiet wisdom—so that he could just go. And so he did eventually go—quietly, nicely, undramatically. And there we were, like frogs on a lily pad in the middle of a stinking, stagnant marsh, avoiding meeting each other's eyes, which would have been like staring at our own newfound ugliness.

After he died I never heard anyone mention him again.

Retrospectively, I believe we all became intimately intertwined in Law's story because it held the infectious, compelling urgency that drew millions of people over several generations to *The Autobiography of Malcolm X*. He was the model prisoner with an eighth-grade education who became professorial in his knowledge of history, and literature, and social science. Listening to Law talk about a plethora of subjects was inspiring, and the virus seemed to be just one way that his mind and body housed the cultural ebbs and flows of American social politics.

Sitting with these difficult and vexing narratives is an occasion for caregivers to democratize the deep feeling of subordination that comes with being a patient. One nurse, in attempting to understand how these poignant influences on the culture emerged at The Space, shared with me the following story of a resident she had known years earlier. It was the incident that transformed her relationship to end-of-life care.

"Death doesn't bother me as much as it used to. I don't take it home with me anymore. I understand now that my job is to help people while they are here and let them go when they are gone. I'm not a religious person, but I was raised Catholic. And I have seen people here go to heaven and hell. It sounds crazy, I know. But I have seen it.

"The story I remember most was a woman named Timie. She had had a hard life, and her stepfather abused her. She also resented her mother a great deal for staying with him. Well, she had turned to the streets, and she got the virus. The day she was actually dying a lot of her friends from the streets came to The Space to be with her. Her mother and stepfather came as well. She was in a coma and her breathing was labored. There were a lot of us in the room when this happened: I was holding onto her leg—I don't know Reiki, but I was holding her leg and trying to relax her body—when all of a sudden, her entire body, her WHOLE BODY, just leapt up and her head turned to face her father and her eyes—they looked like they were literally popping out of her head and she let out this blood-curdling scream right in his face. I have never before, or since, seen anything like it. I had been a very angry, angry person up until that point in my life. And as I continued to hold her leg, I felt as though the anger and the evil and the heavy energy just—I don't know how to explain it—it just sucked right out of me. Just like that.

"I think that she had so much anger in her and she couldn't die with it. I know that there were angels around her protecting her. I could feel them. Other people in the room could feel it too. And she took all of that bad stuff and, at that moment, she spits it at him. And she, in this moment right before her death, she took my anger away too. And she spits that out too. This happened more than seven years ago, and I know that the anger I felt was lifted right out of me. Remember, I am not a religious person, but something happened in there that day. And I have had a different energy ever since. She died minutes after that. And, that stepfather, we never saw him again."

It was unusual for nurses to share stories such as this one. But they were a sobering reminder that patients' experiences have the power to shape the personal and professional trajectories of their caregivers. There were the stories that stretched caregivers' medical understanding. And then there were sublime stores, like Sweet's.

Sweet's story began in 1965 when, as a two-year-old baby, she took a book away from her mother who was reading too slowly. She proceeded to read the book out loud. Her mother, completely aghast, knew Sweet was no ordinary child.

Sweet had a privileged life—equestrian training and debutante balls; slumber parties with prep school girlfriends all wearing matching pajamas; and Sunday afternoon outings to the local ice cream shop with her mom and loving stepdad (he'd adopted her when she was one). She was an inquisitive child: "What *makes* poverty?" and "Why do some suffer more than others?" and "Why aren't people treated equally?" They weren't surprised when the fifteen-year-old, who was graduating from high school two years early, announced, "I want to go to college in New York, in the real world." She went to New York University. And, while there was no question that Sweet was an intellectual gem, less certain was her emotional maturity. She graduated from NYU at nineteen and began law school there. The first time a classmate offered her a treat to take the edge off during exams, she took it.

Cocaine became her friend.

After that, the marginalized folks who peopled the underbelly of lower Manhattan, the very people she intended to help when she became a lawyer, became her suppliers, then her cocaine bedfellows. And before long she found herself pregnant. Unsure of who the father was, and unsure that she had the presence of mind to keep herself alive, let alone a baby, she headed home.

Forty-eight hours after her first obstetric visit she sat blankly, emotionless, wrapping her mind around an HIV diagnosis.

But Sweet committed to getting clean, and staying well, and she invested her time and energy into becoming the mother she knew she was capable of being. She gave birth to a brown-skinned, blue-eyed baby who was coddled and fawned over by her mother and grandparents. The baby, Belle, was healthy, strong, and HIV-negative. The baby's grandparents cared for her punctiliously, and nursed Sweet back to health. One morning Sweet's parents awoke to the baby's cries, and when they went to look for Sweet, she was gone.

I met thirty-one-year-old Sweet four days before she died. She was in and out of consciousness. As soon as we would begin talking, she would drift off, and upon waking, she could not remember what she had said, or meeting me.

She told me that she believed in God and had made bad choices. "It's not too late to make good decisions," I said, but in the four days that I knew her, I was never sure if she heard me.

One day before her death, I went into Sweet's room and found her fast asleep with a crisp grilled cheese sandwich and hot vegetable soup cooling before her. "Sweet," I said. She opened her eyes. "Let's try and eat."

I held her sandwich up to her lips and she took a nibble. Then another. Then another. Her feet were cold and too swollen for socks, and she just wanted to sleep and forget about her pained belly and cold feet. I stroked her hair, and she drifted off to sleep.

The day after that, a nurse stood over my desk where I was doing paper work and told me that I should go see Sweet.

"Okay," I smiled.

"No," she took my pencil out of my hand, "I mean now."

I gave Sweet last rites. She was agitated, unsettled. I read the Bible to her, which seemed to agitate her more. I looked around her room for clues. There was a daily planner, a brush, a bouquet of flowers that had just arrived from her parents in Virginia, and a crime novel. I picked up the novel.

I read, *They found her body on the bank of the East River.* She quieted and listened. A nurses' aide came in. *It won't be the last body they find this way.* The nurses' aide looked at me disapprovingly.

Two chapters in she went to sleep.

More than any resident I have met, Sweet reminds me of myself. We were both born into nurturing families and had attended all-girl schools. We both had a radical and often untamed passion for justice, especially where women and children were concerned. We both sought out and poked people who were too comfortable in their own worlds, and in polite company we met offensive jokes with intolerance and disdain.

Our noisiness and indignation made us obnoxious, but we didn't wait to be told this, because we were our own harshest critics. While I was a research fellow in religion in the environs of Columbia University, Sweet was on a street corner in Harlem, only a couple blocks away.

Stories of banishment and self-imposed exile add breadth to illness narratives in that they democratize class, race, or gendered responses to illness. Sweet's is a story of marginality, spiritual poverty and wealth, and disenfranchisement. To place her narrative amongst more traditional stories of marginalization requires that we confront the universality of suffering. In this confrontation we can each become the subject. And, of course, we can become objects too.

(4.5)

There are some bad stories; stories that beg not to be spoken. There are stories that set our spirits back, that arrest our souls, that threaten to darken our hearts and shrink our humanity.

After you hear those stories, forget them—if you can. But remember the cautionary lesson they bequeath to you.

Dance when you're broken open.
Dance, if you've torn the bandage off.
Dance in the middle of fighting. Dance in your blood.
Dance when you're perfectly free.

—RUMI

5

Losing It

As time went on, I was becoming increasingly consumed by the work, and increasingly heavy-hearted. I was also becoming a better chaplain—more attentive to residents' spiritual wholeness, more spiritually centered in and beyond the community, more present.

And for better or worse, stories followed me everywhere. Two years after I started working at The Space I decided to go to a conference in Hawaii, then enjoy a short reprieve from the obligations of life on the mainland. I wanted and needed to disconnect from the mainland, and to be in a place where I didn't recognize anyone, and no one recognized me. One day, as I was enjoying the luxury of sitting in the hotel lobby, free from the obligation of making conversation, I noticed that the woman next to me was watching me. I pulled a newspaper out of my bag and buried myself in it. But as I stretched my eyes to the right, I could tell that she was still watching me. Unable to enjoy solitude, and fretting the risk of a conversation, I decided to pack up and move to another spot. As I put my paper away she spoke. "Just a beautiful place to sit and relax, isn't it?"

"Yes it is," I responded with a faint smile, as I gathered my bag to move on.

"Is it your first time to Hawaii?" she asked.

"No. Been here before," I replied, my bag now packed and on my lap. "I hope you enjoy your trip." I began to rise.

She waved her arm. "Oh, well, it's only a very short trip," she said. "My partner is attending a conference here at the hotel. We're from California," she smiled, conveying her satisfaction at being a Californian. "Are you here for the conference?" she asked.

"I am," I said mid-stride.

"And you're from …"

"New England," I replied.

"You don't say!" She replied with gusto, and commented that she had attended the local teachers' college in my town. I looked at her blankly. Serendipitously, she was a graduate of the university where I taught, a school so embedded in the periphery of the academy that I could go a lifetime without meeting anyone who was an alumnus of my school, even in the city where the school was located. I scanned the statistical improbability of meeting an alumnus in Hawaii. To conceal that I taught at that university would be like refusing divine mediation.

I had to ride it out.

"I teach there," I said.

"No!" she replied, as if she'd just won the lottery. I asked her what department she was in, and she answered in the form of a question. "English?"

"I am in the English Department," I said, surrendering to the futility in attempting to dodge fate.

She waved her hand animatedly, "Oh, for heaven's sake! Well, that was a million years ago! You're young! But it certainly is a small world."

"That it is," I wavered between walking off and continuing down the rabbit hole.

"My partner is from your neck of the woods in New England, too," she continued. "Maybe you know of her."

"I'm from New York," I replied. "I've only been in New England a short while. It's unlikely that I know her."

"Oh, well, you certainly wouldn't know her. She left a long, long time ago. Her name is Angela. She owned a dance studio in your city."

My mind went to Gregory. If she was a dancer in town, she must know him.

"I don't know an Angela. But she probably knows someone I know. A dancer. Named Gregory—"

She looked up from her beach bag and stared at me.

"Gregory?" she asked.

"Yes," I responded.

"You know Gregory?" Her hands covered her mouth. Then I remembered. Was it possible? Was this the partner of the woman Gregory had told me about as he drifted in and out of consciousness? The woman who had been his mentor and whose son had been tragically killed in a car accident?

As I sunk back into my seat I asked her, "Was your partner's son killed in a car accident?" Her eyes filled with tears. We exchanged information and discovered, that, 5000 miles away from home, I was about to meet the mentor of a patient whose stories about being a Broadway dancer drew me to him every week. Gregory had been estranged from his teacher for many years and for a number of reasons: misunderstandings, money, artistic temperaments.

Later that day, as I listened to his teacher's stories, Gregory began to take on a new life: I was meeting him again, no longer bound by his wheelchair and failing eyes, free from his limited memory and shaking hands. He was leaping across a Broadway stage, performing with Pearl Bailey, dancing for Alvin Ailey, and admonishing young dancers to keep time.

Even 5000 miles away, the stories of this community continued to find me.

That meeting wasn't the only thing that drew me deeper into the spiritual mystery of stories. If you've never been to Hawaii, and you've heard it described as a paradise, you may be inclined to view this as hyperbole. Three years earlier, I'd spent eight weeks doing research at the University of Hawaii; during that trip I had thought paradise might be an understatement, from the breezy seventy-eight degree weather every day, to the excessive number of plumerias that blow from the trees and blanket the sidewalks, to the Hawaiian people who approach every part of their culture—from music, to dance, to food—as sacred. Hawaii is hopeful and healing, beautiful and vibrant. It is what I imagine heaven might be.

So perhaps I wasn't able fully to contextualize alternative thinking about healing and reconciliation at The Space until I spent time at an HIV/AIDS outreach center in Honolulu. The Life Foundation in Honolulu is a non-profit organization founded in 1983 with two goals: to stop the spread of HIV/AIDS and to assist those living with HIV/AIDS. At the time I visited them, the foundation served over 600 HIV-positive people in Hawaii by providing medical, social, and financial support, along with HIV/AIDS education and meals, all in a discrete location. Their services have expanded to accommodate over 700 clients in the last decade. Described as the "front door" to the AIDS care system on Oahu, the Life Foundation provides case workers who assist HIV-positive clients in finding resources and services to meet their special needs. The Life Foundation places a generous amount of advertisements on buses and in public locations, including both the tourist areas and the residential parts of the island.

My first visit to the Life Foundation was incredibly absent of red tape. I called and introduced myself as an HIV/AIDS chaplain from the mainland. I was invited to come in the next day and meet with the public relations director, staffers, and a social worker. New England was never so administratively hospitable and accessible.

I boarded two buses from Waikiki Beach to get to the nondescript corporate office where the Foundation is located. As it turned out, entering the building was only the first step in the journey to find the Life Foundation. As if traveling down Alice in Wonderland's rabbit hole, I took the elevator, then exited the elevator on a floor with surprisingly few doors. Signs to the Life Foundation directed me down a very long corridor, and then another corridor, which ended at a doorway marked "Exit." I was sure I had gone the wrong way, so I retraced my steps and wound up, again, at the "Exit" sign. Upon entering the "Exit" and walking into a dimly lit hallway, I saw another small sign to the Life Foundation. Proceeding down another half-flight of stairs, then through the only available doorway, I was face to face with the entrance. According to the public relations director, the entrance is, in a sense, a metaphor for what the Foundation is: a well-known but discreet and unassuming place, off the beaten path but within twenty-five minutes of one of the most renowned beaches in the world. It was the place where many people living with HIV had sought and received assistance, without also receiving the negative attention that they wished to avoid.

On my second trip to the Life Foundation, the staff invited me to stay for lunch, which was served in their soup kitchen. The soup kitchen was actually a corporate conference room, equipped to accommodate about seventy-five people, with tables set up in rows. About twenty minutes before lunch was to be served, a steady stream of clients, mostly white men, and most of whom appeared to be in couples or acquainted with each other, began to fill up the waiting room outside of the conference area. Four vocal and cheerful men chatted near to where I was seated—an ancient, tattered couch opposite the reception desk. I joined in their conversation, and they graciously included me. When the doors of the conference room opened, feeling a bit like the new kid on the first day of school, I hesitantly asked if I could join them for lunch. They welcomed me with genuine enthusiasm, and two of the men, noting my outsider status, informed me that they were partners who had moved to Hawaii from the mainland only five days earlier and had just taken their first HIV tests. They did not yet know if they were positive, but they had been partners for some time and had chosen to start a new life in a new location before finding out if either one of them—or both of them—had the virus. Both were subdued and anxious. "We just don't know if we have it," said Glen, a strikingly handsome, blond, and boyish man, who was the more outspoken of the two. He stared at me as if his statement was a question, and with genuine concern in his eyes. Glen's partner, Craig, had landed a job on his second day on the island. He would be working at a touristy restaurant in Waikiki as a cook making $7.25 an hour. The other men, all of whom had been on the island for a while, agreed that this was a very good salary.

Volunteers served a lunch of wheat tacos with ground beef, salad, and pistachio ice cream over brownies. The men (there were only men) talked openly about a range of issues, including the high cost of living in Hawaii (balanced by the generous array of social services offered), and the scant red tape involved in accessing support services in Oahu, compared to the mainland. One gentleman gave the example of easily getting his toy-breed dog approved as a service dog to help him cope with an anxiety disorder. This allowed him to bring his dog on the bus, and into stores and restaurants. Another gentleman had lost his Section 8 housing on the Big Island, so he moved to Oahu, where Section 8 housing was easier, he claimed, to acquire, and where more housing options existed.

The most well-known of the men at lunch was David, a highly-revered drag queen in the Honolulu nightclub scene. Until recently, he had not experienced any health problems, but a month before, he started having severe, debilitating pain in his abdomen and gaining a lot of weight. Soon after that he became jaundiced. "By the time my friends took me to the hospital, I had a sore—a huge sore that was like a gaping hole. They gave me morphine and if it hurt that much with morphine, you can't imagine how much it hurt without it." David lifted his shirt to his chin and exposed an elaborate series of bandages. A friend came over as he lifted his shirt and commented on his weight loss. "When I left the hospital," he continued, "I was forty pounds lighter than I was when I went in. They drained fluid from me and the fluid kept draining and draining, which felt wonderful. I could watch my stomach going down."

When I asked David his secret to surviving thirty years with the virus, he shrugged, "Who knows? We all have our preservatives. Mine is Maybelline."

"What about your meds?"

"Never," he said. "I've never taken medication. That stuff kills you. Everyone I know who took meds—and there were hundreds of them—are all dead."

Of course this wasn't a medical statistic, but it was his unfiltered recollection.

"What about alternative medicine?" I asked

"What alternative? I've lived my life and when it's my time, it's my time. I will never trade one poison for another." I inquired further about David's self-care practices. "I bathe in the Pacific Ocean. I wake up in paradise every day. This place makes me well."

Interviews with staff members echoed a similar feeling about the healing nature of Hawaiian culture and lifestyle and a general ethos undergirding native Hawaiian responses to illness. One case manager in Native Hawaiian Services described the approach to HIV as "trying to use or reestablish traditional values among those who have lost their sense of connection to what it means to be Hawaiian, and the spirituality that grounds our culture.

"The main problem we face," the case manager continued, "is lack of education about HIV, and with native Hawaiians, the knowledge is even poorer than among the general population."

Although it is not the primary mode of contracting the infection for native Hawaiians, homosexual relationships remain an issue in need of more open dialogue. Among natives, the case worker explains, "people who are *Mahoos*, who are gay, have a place of honor in Hawaiian communities because they are considered to be more spiritual—to possess the spirit of both a male and a female, thus they are more divine." Even given this, "native Hawaiians are not so liberal about sexuality, because most are Christian. So working within these spaces can be tricky."

The Life Foundation created the "No Shame" campaign to deal with issues that are specific to being native Hawaiian and HIV-positive. Ideally, the "No Shame" campaign might encourage people living in rural areas to go to a hospital if they are sick, even though they fear the mainstream medical establishment "managing" their illness, or fear shaming their families. "Interestingly," the case worker notes, "most people who are HIV-positive do eventually disclose their HIV status and their sexual preferences to their families and they are never—*ever*—put out." While the family and even the local community may know a loved one's HIV status, the medical establishment—including doctors—are considered the medical outsiders. "At the time of death, family members will fight not to have 'HIV/AIDS-related illness' listed as the cause of death. Who are they now hiding this from, since they have all come to terms with this? Once they are over the shock of the diagnosis, they don't want this to be the legacy that their loved one leaves. It isn't about the 'public,' it's about the pride of the community."

I returned from Hawaii calmer, more peaceful, healthier, and refreshed. I had been the recipient of hospitality, generosity, warmth, and beauty, and felt renewed in my approach to HIV/ AIDS care.

Upon my return, New England was cold, sterile, unwelcoming. I was greeted by a co-worker who was a thirty-six-year-old woman trapped in a job she had come to despise, and working with a cast of characters who devalued her work and found her insufferable. Because she had years of experience as a social worker, but was not academically credentialed, she could not find another job. She was perpetually steeped in the drama of a reality star on steroids. She caught me as I walked in:

> Oh my God, I'm so glad you're back. You would never believe what has been going on here . . . first of all Cassie *peed* in her chair during women's group, I mean *urine*. Then Bonita tells her she's nasty and so I turn to the group and tell them that I happen to agree—that Cassie *is* being nasty—and that maybe we should ask her to leave, and call maintenance on her way back to her room.

Where is Cassie now? I asked.

I hear she's sitting in the rec room in her peed-up pants! She is looking for attention and acting out and she's gonna get attention alright.

I'm pretty sure she couldn't help it, I offered.

She has got to take some responsibility. Look at *me*, for example. Last week I find out from my doctor that I have a hole in my back—I was probably born with it— and I can barely walk now. Look how I walk [she wobbles past me awkwardly, then wobbles back]. Not to mention my blood pressure is sky high and I don't even have any feeling in my hands from carpal tunnel. Touch my hand. Not there, *here*. You see that?

(I don't see anything.)

When you touch it the pain shoots right up my arm and across my back! And that started with another thing that I can't really talk about.

Sorry you can't talk about it. (I started to walk away.)

Well, what happened was, you know that new social service guy? He made a pass at me. And not just a pass. Fine. I'll tell you. He actually opened his pants—his pants!— and tried to expose himself. Right in front of me! *And* he has been trying to touch me, too.

(I stood before her with an inappropriately blank look on my face. I could not imagine how I should look when a case worker, trained in sexual misconduct, shared an incident of sexual assault as an afterthought.)

That wouldn't be so bad [*really?*], except when I told the head nurse about it she pulled me into her office BY MY EAR! And left a bruise! [*She points to her unscathed left ear.*] Do you see? Right there! [*She points to it again.*] So of course I went to the executive director and told her what happened and she wrote up some kind of report, and as a result of that report I get called in and penalized by the supervisor who exposed himself. For insubordination! All this time my head is pounding and my lungs feel like they are collapsing. And as if that wasn't enough, my liver hurts. I mean REALLY hurts! [*How do you know your liver hurts?*] Actually, it has to do with my cholesterol. Oh God, don't even get me started. [*I don't intend to....*] I'd love to get out of this place right now, but my night vision is so bad that I have to wait for my husband to pick me up, and he is just recovering from his accident—his carjacking. [*He carjacked someone?*] Are you kidding? Are you? HE was carjacked ... These, well, I'll just say thugs ... They were actually black people, to be honest. There, I said it: they were blacks. I'm not saying that has anything to do with it. Obviously it doesn't .... [*Obviously.*] They actually pulled him out of his car, looted his car, and when they were done they put him BACK in the driver's seat and rolled him—the whole car—off a cliff.

I was deeply devoted—tactically—to avoiding any comment that might serve as a prompt.

"I appreciate your desire to share with me and I hope talking about it was helpful," I said, "but I have quite a bit of work to do. I think I have to go for now. And I will certainly pray for you."

I spent a good part of my day trying to figure out how to minimize these interactions, searching for the words to bridge concern with calculated distance, trying to figure out how to turn such encounters into spiritual opportunities. While I recognized that staffers had stories too, I had reached "story saturation." Despite the Hawaiian reprieve, despite my prayerfulness and the genuine joy I found in serving, despite my passion for working with and listening to people living with HIV/AIDS, I was burning out.

(5.5)

In a myth circulated in rural villages scattered throughout various corners of the African continent, but popularized in South Africa—and in the west by the dangerous humor of the play *The Book of Mormon*—it is believed that men with AIDS can be cured by having sexual relations with a female virgin, not excluding infants. At the start of the twenty-first century, the "virgin cure," as it is commonly known, resulted in South Africa having the highest rates of child rape worldwide. Before its current iteration relating to the AIDS virus, this myth and similar ones have a long history in Europe and Asia as well, and they speak to the medicinal, social, and political import of gender inequality in cultural narratives— particularly the role of these narratives in justifying the subordination of women and girls.

I mention this to demonstrate that there are always moments when medical and social culture must seek entrance into the fabric of the mythological narratives in communities. Even decades later, many cultures have to stretch their popular understanding of illness discourse in order to make space for this modern and medically extraterrestrial disease. The ever-present disjuncture between traditional practices and the scientific community have often resulted in a failure—on both sides—to effectively curb the spread of HIV and AIDS.

I know that in my time at The Space, I encountered many residents who, frustrated with the medical establishment, sought to construct their own "remedies." One resident, an obsessive cornstarch-eater, recounted that when she was a child, her mother and grandmother—many of her kinfolk, but mostly the women—ate cornstarch as a cure-all. As a child she was told that the habit started with pregnancy, but childless women ate it as well. She tried it and was immediately addicted. When I asked her to describe the taste she said, "It's better than any food I can think of. It's sweet-like." She continued, "And this is the thing: I feel like I just can't eat enough of it. I've been eating it for years now. *And it helps me.*" She went on to say that she could do without drugs or cigarettes, but she couldn't live without cornstarch.

According to Dr. W. Clay Jackson, amylophagia, or the practice of consuming purified starch, is a form of pica, the compulsive digestion of non-food materials such as coal or dirt that is linked to iron deficiencies. While it appears among patients worldwide, it is particularly prevalent among rural African American women, and it is believed to be a complex behavioral phenomenon resulting from the interplay of biochemical, hematological, psychological, and cultural factors.[1]

And as I listen to doctors talk about pica and HIV/AIDS patients during rounds and think about the "virgin cure"—that most deviant explication of child rape—I'm aware that where the medical community falls short, dangerous cultural narratives can step in.

That is why medicine is most effective when it is culturally anthropological; medicine thrives when it is connected to stories.

---

1. Jackson, "Amylophagia Presenting as Gestational Diabetes," 649.

Don't grieve. Anything you lose comes round in another form.

—RUMI

6

Questions without Answers

The loud explosion was followed by whiteness blanketing my windshield—then clouds of smoke billowing around my windows.

I drove slowly, and my headlights, cutting through the thick smoke and darkness, revealed a terrifically mangled car on the opposite side of the road. As my car cut through a second wave of smoke, I could see that the vehicle looked as though it had been sawed in half. Then I became aware that, other than the loud explosion, there was deafening silence, and not a single soul around.

Suddenly, a woman appeared out of nowhere shouting, "Get them out! It's going to blow up! Jesus, get them out!" I made my way by foot to the opposite side of the street and looked for any sign of life around me. The passenger side of the car was wholly crumpled, as if it were made of tin foil. Then, through the rolls of billowing smoke, I saw a disheveled man stumbling up the street, apparently severely disoriented, or drunk. The smoke was suddenly penetrated by the glaring headlights of the two cars involved in the accident, each facing the other about thirty feet apart. The stumbling man was bobbing in and out of view.

"Is anyone hurt?" he slurred. I looked through the driver side window of the mangled car. A man was slumped over the driver seat with blood all around his face. I looked down and saw that his hand was severed. I walked around to the passenger side and realized that the seat was empty, and that the door had been opened. The passenger, I believe, was the woman screaming in the street. In the back of the car was a bloodied young girl moaning lightly.

"Get them out for God's sake!" The woman in the street yelled."The car is going to blow!"

Two truckers emerged through the smoke and went to work on the door entrapping the girl.

"Pull! Pull!" As they tried to pry the doors open to get the trapped passengers out, I thought, *what happens after this car explodes in our faces?* I leaned in the window close to the bloody girl in the back seat.

"What is your name?"

She rolled her head to the side and whispered. "Jessica."

"Jessica, you're okay." Blood dripped from a piece of glass lodged in her forehead.

Where is the ambulance? The truckers unhinged part of the front door, but stepped back when they saw the man's distorted limb. The man with the severed hand rolled out of the passenger side door and lay down on the sidewalk.

I touched Jessica's forehead.

Her head rolled toward me. "*Listen*," she said in a whisper. I leaned in. "Look under the seat. There is an envelope filled with money." I found the envelope. "That's my son's Christmas money. Please, put it away." I folded the envelope and put it in her side pocket. "Now find my keys," she whispered. I found her keys under the car seat. I put them in her pocket too.

I heard the chaos around me—a pop, a scream, the muffled voices of frightened people. Jessica's face was so covered in pumping blood, her hair so matted, that I could not remember what she had looked like a couple minutes before.

"I'm going to sleep now," she said. She took a deep breath and exhaled. A rush of blood came out of her neck. I tried to stop it with her jacket. She seemed to have stopped breathing. I leaned forward to check for a pulse and felt nothing but clamminess. I tilted my head through the window to give her mouth-to-mouth resuscitation, but I couldn't reach her. My hands were clammy and heavy, as if covered in molasses.

I tried to pull out of the car and realized that my hand was caught in a death grip with hers. "JESSICA," I shouted, "COME BACK. *YOUR SON NEEDS YOU!*"

She opened her eyes slightly and drew a shallow breath through bloodied lips.

"Keep your eyes open. You have to stay awake."

At that moment, the flashing ambulance lights penetrated the haze, and as the paramedics and firemen descended upon the scene I drifted to the sidewalk, then to my car. And then I drove away, a smattering of blood on my steering wheel, watching the flashing lights in my rear-view mirror.

I showered, then walked aimlessly around my apartment for hours. I called the local university hospital and discovered that everyone from the accident had been taken there. At about one in the morning, I could no longer bear not knowing. I got dressed and went down to the hospital, needing to know if Jessica was alive. I parked at a meter outside the hospital as I had done every week for four years, but on this night, a night guard, a guy I had never seen before, told me that I should pull my car into the lot, free of charge, so that he could watch the car for me, "however long *this* will take," he said. I didn't know what "this" was, but I thanked him and told him that my car would be fine at a meter. He said okay, and promised me that he would keep an eye on it while I "did what I had to do."

I looked at him curiously and made haste to the emergency room.

As I approached the main entrance of the hospital, there was a double-parked car, and in the front passenger seat there was a woman who appeared to be in distress. A hospital worker had come out to help her and stood alongside the driver, who, I assume, was a relative. As I passed by, the woman in distress gasped uncomfortably, then looked up at me. Her eyes, which were sleepy, flew wide open, and her head turned as she followed my movement into the hospital. The people beside her—the hospital worker and the family member—followed me with their eyes as well. Suddenly she stretched her hand in my direction. I was frightened, and I kept walking.

I told the desk attendant who I was looking for, and she told me to go back to see the girl, Jessica. As I made my way to the rear of the emergency ward, I passed an elderly man stretched out on a gurney. As I passed, he made direct eye contact with me. Then he, like the woman outside, stretched his hand out to me. My uncertainty had turned to trepidation, and in that moment I couldn't wrap my head around my sense of communion with a string of strangers.

I walked on.

I didn't see Jessica yet. But I passed another gentleman who looked as if he had also been in an accident. I tilted my head and looked at him. He tilted his head and looked at me. He pulled his hand from under the covers, but I looked away, fully afraid. I felt an inexplicable present-ness around me and realized that I felt more awake, more conscious, than I remembered ever having been in my life. I felt as though I was looking into all of the people around me. It seemed my hearing was crisper, my vision sharper, very much like the night Omez died, and the universe seemed to be coming apart and reassembling around me.

Jessica was in the farthest corner of the emergency room and she was in and out of consciousness. I approached her bed. "Jessica," I said.

"You're here," she said, then to her nurse, "This is her."

"Well," he said, thoughtfully, "we've been hearing all evening about the angel in her car window. Is that you?"

"No," I said. I noticed a young black man with braids for the first time. He was standing on the other side of the bed.

The gaping red wound in her forehead was now fastened together with thick, black thread, like a crude quilt. I was examining them closely when the police arrived.

They immediately began to ask who had been at the scene. Jessica's boyfriend stared at them blankly, as if he didn't understand the question. "Do you remember what happened?" The officer asked, with arrested empathy. "The man," she whispered, "The man hit us." She turned her head to the side and closed her eyes.

The officer looked at me. "I arrived after the accident," I told him.

"Who was driving when you approached the car?" he asked.

"I didn't approach the other man's car," I say. "I only approached theirs. The other woman was driving."

Jessica's eyes shot open. "No she wasn't. Pepe was driving." The officer looked at me, then back at Jessica. The guy with the severed hand—whose name, it appears was Pepe, had been in the driver's seat when I approached the car. But, as I thought about it, his severed hand had been on the passenger side. I never learned the back story, but imagine: changing seats and leaving your hand behind.

The officer looked back at Jessica. "None of you were wearing seat belts. You're lucky to be alive." Jessica closed her eyes again. He noted something on his notepad and looked back at me. "Anything else?"

"No," I responded.

"Thank you for your time," he said, shutting his notepad.

That night, the car crash, the hand, the messy brush with mortality took a new emotional toll on me. As I became more involved in chaplaincy and more attuned to a spiritual calling to help the sick, human *need* seemed to find me—or I it—everywhere I turned. Over the years, the feeling of purposefulness was now a deeply comfortable fatigue.

As I reflect on it now, I am reminded of my first trip to Europe as a graduate student. I was traveling from London to Liverpool to attend a conference, then back to London to visit family. I didn't own a suitcase with wheels, so I took a large duffle bag with me, filled with clothes and an outrageous number of books that I thought I'd be able to read both on the plane and on the trains here and there. In addition to the heavy books, which were causing awful soreness in my shoulders, I picked up a host of knickknacks along the way—a bell for mom's bell collection and a University of Liverpool sweatshirt for my sister—and my load got heavier and heavier. I was traveling with a friend who had warned me about the error of my ways. So in order to disprove her suggestion that I needed a suitcase with wheels, I was now forced, in addition to my suffering, to *act* as if my bag was not heavy. My sophisticated solution to the heavy-bag dilemma was to rip out and throw away each page of my books as I read, as if the weight of a dozen book pages would make a difference. By the time my friend and I were heading back to the States, I had every reason to think I'd probably done short-term but poignant damage to my aching and travel-weary arms.

Not knowing how to avoid becoming overwhelmed by my exhaustion and despondency—and needing to keep up with teaching and chaplaincy without any one thing being compromised—I buried a great deal of distress and frustration inside, carrying it like that crazy duffle bag, letting go of a page here and there, but not dealing efficiently with the root of the problem. Carrying stories everywhere made me feel less guilty, less conflicted about the profound distance between my personal life and the lives of residents at The Space. What kind of person was I if I could bear witness to painful suffering and then partake gluttonously in elaborate meals with friends? Insincere? Apathetic? Cold-hearted? There was something about listening to residents' complicated stories, then gleefully cutting up with a girlfriend on the phone, that made me feel like a charlatan. Which reality was true? How can heartfelt emotions be pocketed as easily as shifting location? What was real? Essentially, what did I owe the residents when I wasn't with them?

After Christmas my fatigue turned to frustration when The Space welcomed a new director of Social Services, who was to be my supervisor. He came to The Space from a geriatric facility and had limited experience with people with AIDS, urban populations, people with a history of addiction, and (I assume people of color). In his interactions with residents he would tuck his hands deeply into the pockets of his tidily pressed Dockers and tilt his head, with an expression of muted disinterest, while residents would chat him up about myriad issues. "How are you, Michael?" he would address said resident, with a look that suggested more courtesy than concern. I'd lean against the nurses' station with residents and watch.

"So you the new social worker?" Michael would respond. "Good, I got some questions for you about my Social Security, 'cause I haven't been getting my mail, and since I been here no one can tell me what happened to my checks …"

At the end of Michael's long soliloquy, the supervisor would inform him to "see Diane about that. Have a good day, now." The resident would stare at the supervisor blankly as he walked away. Even if the resident continued to stare at him with uncertainty, he would—with a level of comfort beyond that warranted by the situation—walk away. He would move gingerly to the next resident.

"How are you, Mildred?"

"Oh, not so good today," Mildred would say, looking up at him woefully from her wheelchair. "My hip is paining me something awful, and they been telling me for months that it needs to be operated on, but no surgery gets scheduled. Don't look like nothing is gonna happen. Look like the pain just getting worse and worse, 'til I can't barely stand it."

"Well, you have a good day, Mildred," and the supervisor would continue down the hall, delivering pleasantries.

The supervisor was part of the young blood that mixed with old world-weary blood and together came up with the time clock, among other bean-counting measures. The longer I watched the supervisor's behavior among the residents, the more he reflected to me the way all big corporations have the opportunity to earn consumer trust with integrity, or crush the will of dispirited workers—whichever suits their fancy.

The supervisor had been at The Space six weeks when I was called into his office. His hands were stuffed awkwardly into his pockets, even though he was sitting. "I was reviewing your time sheet, and I noted that you only did eight hours last week … not the required ten hours."

"Okay," I met his blank stare.

"Is there something you'd like to say—some explanation you'd like to offer for this?" He smiled slightly. Though my expression remained vacant, I felt my blood pressure rising. I had ten minutes before I had to leave. In my other life, I was now the director of a graduate program in women's studies; I was preparing for the release of my first book, and leaving in a few days to present a paper at an international AIDS conference. More importantly, only a few feet away, residents were waiting for "lost" Social Security checks and the opportunity to schedule well overdue hip replacements.

He continued, "I'm looking at what has been clocked. According to the time clock—"

"I don't *clock* funerals."

"And I don't read minds."

"I'm sorry—I didn't realize this conversation was about … Did you have any other questions?" I asked dryly.

"You just have to understand … the time clock … it's our only way of knowing for sure that people are working *and not goofing off*—"

"Did you say '*goofing off?*'"

He shrugged, "Well, yes, goofing off."

I stood up, "You should pay me for the eight hours that were punched in. Are we all set?"

"Actually, we're not all set. One day it seems you forgot to punch out, so the clock … See, it's important that we're all on board in terms of sticking to the rules."

I stood still, still meeting his empty stare with my own empty stare.

"Is that it?" I asked.

I was taken aback by his clock preoccupation when several residents, on *his* watch, were missing benefits, searching aimlessly for lost relatives, struggling to get their GEDs, waiting on rides for dialysis, and trying to get on transitional housing lists.

Then, there was the clock.

"I think I'll refer this to the executive director," he suggested. "We can get her perspective."

I got up and left.

One week later I was called into a meeting with the executive director, the head nurse, and the supervisor. The director had a deep appreciation for the spiritual care program we were building at The Space, including the first palliative care protocol "guidebook" in the facility's history and a growing crew of spiritual care volunteers representing different religious traditions and denominations within them. The executive director looked embarrassed and avoided eye contact with me as she commented "broadly" on the importance of the clock. She and I had a warm, collegial relationship; this type of interaction was without precedent, but consistent with the shifting trends in longterm care. "Your office is being moved to the basement to save space on the main floor," the supervisor wadded with a grin.

I went downstairs to take a look at the space to which I had been moved, a windowless, cold corner of half-finished basement with a dusty plywood desk and no phone. The desk drawers were locked and there were no keys. It was freezing. When I went back upstairs, the maintenance guy offered to move my boxes, shook his head, and draped his arm around me as we walked.

I retreated to the nurses' station to chart for the day. A nurse, one of many who depended upon spiritual care as necessary to wellness, patted my back and sighed. A second nurse was more animated. She barked an expletive as she filled medicine cups, and within a few hours, several reported to the director that they needed the chaplain on the floor. I considered this "demotion" to be turning into a blessing: it had taken years to build mutual trust with the nurses and doctors (the stories I shared with them lent insight, if not answers), but because the supervisor was immovable, I became a laughable "bag lady," lugging all of my supplies—bibles, communion, clipboards, and rosaries—in a huge bag, like a traveling saleswoman.

One day, as I was dragging my bag behind me to the front of the facility, I noticed the maintenance crew receiving a large shipment of boxes at the front door. And more boxes. There were boxes upon boxes upon boxes, and by the time they were done there were about twelve medium-sized lightweight boxes neatly stacked against the wall.

"My Christmas presents?" I asked.

"You wish, Chap! Naw, these are for a resident. New dude named Gerome. So many of them we have to open them—make sure it's up and up."

A security guard with a box cutter opened the first box and pulled out hand lotion, then soap, then a wax lip balm. He opened the second and unearthed a nail polish set and bubble bath. Beauty product after beauty product. All were from Avon. They invited me to come along as they delivered the shipment to Gerome. I had not met Gerome, and when we arrived at his room we were greeted by a dark-skinned black man of about sixty years sitting upright in his bed, wearing just a sleeveless t-shirt and playing solitaire. Gerome was morbidly obese and only able to get around in a scooter. In a deep, gravelly voice with no affect he said, "Good. My stuff is here."

"Why you need all of this girl stuff, man?" the security guard asked.

"Just need it. Like it. Sometimes I share it." He flipped a card out of his hand onto the bed.

"All right, well, just watch yourself," said the guard. "Looks shady to me."

Whether it was shady or not I can't say, but this I know for sure: Gerome was the most prolific Avon representative I've ever met. Residents would buy things, often spending more money than they could afford to spend. Behind the nurses' station, nurses and nurses' aides could be seen thumbing through Avon catalogs, then heading to his room with a pen. Boxes came, then more boxes. With money in his pocket, Gerome would ride his scooter up the block to the donut shop, where he would wait in line at the drive through, sandwiched between two cars, and order a dozen donuts. Then he'd ride back to The Space with them and hole up in his room eating donuts.

The Avon sales went on for three months, at which point social services caught wind that he was running a business. Was it actually a violation of house rules? On what grounds could he be prevented from exploring a private (and pre-existing) interest? In the end, he was told that if he was well enough to run a business then he was well enough to leave The Space. The nurses and nurses' aides were told that if they ordered from him they would be penalized. They said—and it is true—that it just isn't easy to find Avon representatives anymore.

Around this time, and despite the levity that such instances provided, I started to feel stories bleeding into other parts of my life. During a perfectly lovely dinner conversation with my women's club or with colleagues, I might find myself talking about a patient's death, then trying to focus on *not* doing that. I was not oblivious to the impact this had on listeners—I often regretted mentioning such things almost as soon as I registered the discomfort on the listeners' faces—but I didn't know how *not* to talk about it, how to move people living with HIV/AIDS *out* of their banishment without "showcasing" HIV/AIDS in places where it was inappropriate or unwelcome.

Uncertainty evolved into a sadness that reared its head at night when, mulling around a large, deafeningly quiet apartment in a big city, I would think in endless loops about what I'd seen that day. The flip side of foreboding nights was morning enthusiasm about the endless opportunities to make a difference in someone's life. I owed them a chaplain who was always bright-eyed, energetic, and optimistic. One week I'd come up with a plan for fundraising that would introduce a larger community of donors to our facility. I could get musical instrument donations, and have students from a local conservatory give free lessons to residents (couldn't I?). I could find Resident A's long lost daughter, and reunite Resident B with his mother. I came to understand this boundless eagerness as my very own "savior complex," a feeling that I was able, and required, to fix every dilemma, every problem, every "wrong" that I observed. If a resident had cold feet, I felt responsible for getting socks. Rather than wait for someone else to provide assistance, I simply set out to fix everything myself. Before long, I'd bound myself to a never-ending list of after-work errands and follow-up phone calls. In my life as a professor, my "work day" never ended, as there were always papers to grade and lecture to prepare. I was beginning to see that I was engaged in two jobs without nine-to-five boundaries. I had become a full-time full-timer. There was always work to be done.

There is one obvious and unavoidable problem with the "savior complex:" despite the compulsion to meet everyone's needs we cannot, in any literal sense, rescue everyone, and we are not meant to. The list of "things," material and intangible, needed by people who, in this case, are not entirely self-sufficient, is everlasting; it will never get shorter. Moreover, the things they request often are mere Band-Aids to disguise their real needs. One resident repeatedly begged for reading glasses, because—for reasons that were unclear to me—she had not received a prescription during her doctor's visits. I bought her an old pair that I hoped would suffice for a while. But I soon discovered that this woman was suffering from very early onset dementia, and her true problem was that she could not remember what she had read. The truth is, there was always a need behind the need.

Attempting to fix all of the problems extracts energy and intent away from the recipient of kindness and onto the caregiver: instead of trying to track down a lost check, it would have been better to spend that energy helping residents to seek answers to their own questions. Such a mindset not only enforced accountability, but it also allowed me to empower residents to advocate for themselves, while relieving myself of an array of tasks that drew energy away from spiritual care.

As I was working my way through these boundaries, I started to experience a feeling of separateness from God. I was a chaplain whose work was now about "doing" but not "experiencing." I felt as though I had a choice: I could invest energy in doing what needed to be done or I could be still, reflective, and prayerful. I chose the former. I realize now that although the residents had a chaplain who was getting a lot done for them (and with them), I was not a quiet presence. They often saw me as busy, rushing—making lists and scratching things off—rather than focused, in the present, and aware. I know now that the answer was not always to fill the needs of the sick, but, rather, simply to hear their needs, and to provide a venue for residents to process their feelings. This charge is difficult for those of us who are prescriptive, solution-centered doers. But without quiet prayerfulness the deeper question that was behind all of their needs—*Why am I suffering?*—could never be answered.

During these times, when I turned away from prayerful quietness, I would seek out other "vices" to fill the gap that was left. The vice, for me, was food. It started with returning home from work exhausted and showering to wash off all of the weight of the day, then opting for a big bowl of cereal for dinner, followed by some chips before bed. On nights when I felt ambitious, I would stop to pick up a pizza. I'd strip off my clothes and sit at the table in front of the television, with an entire pizza stretched out before me. I would eat one slice, then another, then another, hardly noticing how much I consumed during a half-hour sitcom. The meal was over only when the program was done, which was generally half a pizza pie and a bottle of orange soda later. I was doing just what I wanted to do with my one, healthy life: sit in my apartment alone, in my underwear, and eat unlimited amounts of pizza. Some nights it would be McDonald's, which always left me feeling much more sluggish and regretful than pizza. Nevertheless, the point was that greasy fast food had become, in my mind, something that I earned, something to help me cope with the difficult work scenarios that I was negotiating regularly. I had become a food addict.

Too busy, and without the physical or emotional energy to exercise, I gained seventeen pounds in the first year. I was answering my phone less and less, not because I was sad, but because I no longer had patience for "ordinary" problems. One friend missed a big sale and therefore wouldn't be able to buy her fourteenth Coach bag. Another friend couldn't decide whether to go to Jamaica or Turks and Caicos on vacation. And yet another couldn't get her husband to stop eating egg salad sandwiches before dinner. To compensate for my dismissiveness towards my friends, I'd throw "apology" dinner parties about once a month, feasts of five-layer lasagna, parmesan-coated arugula, Italian bread smothered in butter and garlic, and chocolate martinis.

By my second year at The Space I had gained twenty-seven pounds.

The nurses had come to depend on me; the residents trusted me. And administrators and doctors included me in discussions and meetings that wouldn't generally include the chaplain. The spiritual life at The Space was vibrant, with a rich variety of services, support groups, and, finally, an end-of-life "program" that assured each patient would receive comprehensive palliative support. Despite this, with the extra weight I gained, I had very little energy, and in a year and a half, I'd survived two bouts of treatment for Norwegian scabies—aggressive opportunistic mites that burrow into the skin, and that are more commonly contracted among residents who were previously homeless. My frustration with the unfairness of life would bare fangs when I was talking to friends pleading with me to take weekend trips to New York— whole weekends—to have uninterrupted days of shopping at Louis Vuitton. It wasn't their gratuitous consumption that bothered me; it was the undertone of entitlement: *I go to work, therefore I am entitled to elaborate gifts.* Well, isn't everyone? Even as people of faith, everyone around me seemed to be living in willful disregard for the calling of every religious tradition: to live unassumingly, to give generously and hold onto nothing that thwarts our path to truth. I was far from being a religious zealot; in fact, I was admittedly entirely without answers. I didn't even have the tools to heal myself; nevertheless, I was self-righteous in my conviction that at least I was asking the difficult questions and doing the hard work.

Wasn't I?

And what is wellness anyway? Wasn't Gandhi devoted to chastity practices that have become the prosaic musings of psychoanalysts? Didn't Martin Luther King deal with stress by compulsive chainsmoking and, before him, wasn't Martin Luther the poster boy for joyous inebriation?

Burnout, fatigue, and compounded stress are common phenomena among people who work with the ill and dying. One medical student whom I met at The Space informed me that she was ill-prepared for the severity of frustration she felt as she learned the limits of her ability to help. She also noted that she was previously unaware of the high levels of suicide among medical students, and she attributed some of these problems to physicians meeting stonewalls when attempting to fully serve their patients.

One study suggests that, for nurses, the profession holds the appeal of helping others through the exercise of professional autonomy and teamwork, "only to be deprived of both by [colleagues] who see nursing roles less imaginatively." Moreover "work overload, uncooperative patients, criticism, negligent coworkers, lack of support from supervisors and difficulty with physicians were associated with stress in nurses."[1]

Over and over again I asked myself, *what does it mean to serve well?* Perhaps, I thought, it means we must find joy in whatever task we are engaged in at the moment, thus freeing us to do even the most mundane tasks joyfully. If the task you are engaging in is something in which you refuse to find pleasure, then what are you feeling instead? Hurriedness? Annoyance? Absence of thought altogether? Ultimately, how are any of these more useful than joy?

In *From Sadness to Pride: Seven Common Emotional Experiences of Caregiving,* Barry Jacobs, a clinical psychologist in Pennsylvania, recounts his experiences with two spouses dealing with the deaths of their wife and husband, respectively. The husband who was dealing with watching his wife die after a long bout with cancer was visibly shaken, and barely able to communicate with the hospital staff without tearfulness, sobbing endlessly over her bed. The woman in the next room was losing her husband to heart failure, and he noted that she sat by his side stylishly dressed and "tight-lipped," showing very little emotion. Once Jacobs became more involved in their cases, he learned that the husband had failed to care for his wife during much of her cancer battle, and had virtually neglected her in the throes of her illness. The "tight-lipped" woman, on the other hand, had experienced a solid marriage with her husband, having experienced forty years of loving devotion. As Jacobs explains, "The wife's lack of expression during

1. Moffitt, "The Relationship Between Burnout and Self-Esteem in Nurses," 2.

his decline stemmed not from lack of caring but from its opposite—the assurance that they had said and exhibited their love for
one another so truly over so long a time that nothing more needed
to be added now. The prospect of death had only brought them to
a wordless contemplation of the deeply felt connection between
them."[2] As one bioethics consultant described it, family caregivers of dying patients find themselves in the most vulnerable and
fragile positions they have probably ever occupied, "with a level of
physical exertion and emotional endurance probably unrivaled by
any other experience they are likely to encounter." [3]

Holly Whitcomb, a United Church of Christ minister, noted,
in regards to balancing grief ministry and everyday life,

> My care of small children, my care of a congregation, my
> care of a physician husband with a demanding schedule
> of his own was too much for me to handle. I eventually
> developed recurrent migraines in which I would tem-
> porarily lose half my vision. (Was God trying to tell me
> that I was literally losing sight of what was important?)
> My own self-protection told me I could never work hard
> enough or please enough people. I allowed myself to live
> fearfully and remained outer directed, rarely allowing
> the Angel of Grace to draw near. I was God's cheerleader
> who had lost her cheer.[4]

Hospital workers, including spiritual caregivers in medical settings, deal with highly atypical workplace stress, including
managing illness, complicated workloads, understaffing, unrelenting timetables, hierarchies, negotiating patients and families, and
coping with death. In addition, the increasing patient volume and
administrative red tape of many hospitals may depersonalize the
environment, leaving workers feeling isolated, drained, ineffective,
and discouraged. These feelings may also be expressed as apathy,
a decrease in feelings of self-worth, withdrawal, or absenteeism.

---

2. Levine, ed., *Always on Call*, 110.
3. Levine, ed., *Always on Call*, 111.
4. Everist, ed., *Ordinary Ministry, Extraordinary Challenges*, 36.

Failure to acknowledge, address, or relieve the sources of stress results in workers who suffer burnout.

Early on in my chaplaincy it became clear to me that observing the end-of-life process requires a lot of the caregivers and loved ones. If people were in pain as they were dying, then I allowed myself to experience pain with them, to the point where I would physically connect with their pain. I would feel drained after touching them, deeply drawn into their suffering, physically and emotionally bound to their experiences. Inasmuch as this experience was the richest human bonding I have ever been blessed to experience, I also had to make peace with the reality that someone else's death is not about me. It is an intimate process that they are engaged in, paced and dictated by their intimate relationship with the universe or their God. We have the power to love, to care, to touch, and to enrich our own mortality by being with the living in all stages, and finding space to celebrate the absolute divinity of each season.

Several months after the Christmas car accident, I was driving near The Space. I was thinking about spending Easter in New York with a priest in Harlem who'd nurtured my soul since I was a girl. I pulled up to a streetlight and was distracted by a hip-hop rhythm vibrating the car next to me. I looked over and saw a young Hispanic girl in the back seat swaying to the rhythm. She moved so freely because she was not wearing a seatbelt. At once, she turned and looked at me. There was a long deep scar across her forehead. It was Jessica, the girl who had been in the car accident that night in December.

There are, I discovered, no easy answers.

(6.5)

(On Rumi)

Rumi was a Muslim theologian, teacher, and poet. While he is now recognized as one of the greatest poets of all time, and his talent was apparent from his youth, it was his meeting a man named Shams—who was himself a lonely sojourner looking for a traveling companion—that changed the course of his life. Their friendship became the soil on which Rumi's spiritual and intellectual prowess was cultivated. One night, Shams went outside and never returned; it is rumored that he was killed by Rumi's son.

Rumi's grief over the loss of his friend resulted in over 70,000 poems over almost three decades. His reckoning with his loss was finally laid to rest with the following words:

> Why should I seek? I am the same as
> He. His essence speaks through me.
> I have been looking for myself!

We are all, when we try to get inside the stories of others, seeking to pry open our own hearts, and souls, and minds.

Don't grieve. Anything you lose comes round in another form.

—RUMI

7

Conclusion

I am shamelessly thinking about brushing my teeth with my three-year-old daughter's toothbrush, and even thinking about the soft bristles against my teeth. I'm whispering a morning prayer to myself as I grip the tiny handle and pull a draw open to find a hair comb. I stop and remember. I rip open the shower curtain and see the mommy toothbrush in the shower caddy where I left it the night before. I toss her tiny toothbrush in the garbage and peel open a new one for her. As I reach for the big girl toothbrush, my one-year-old, who has wrapped herself around my leg, is suspended mid-air, laughing. I can't remember what I was praying about, because I'm now aware that any minute, my one-year-old daughter's laughter will turn to tears as I begin to comb her hair.

My three-year-old enters the bathroom. She wants to wear her ballet slippers to pre-school. And a princess dress. And a tiara. And lipstick. I suggest that we compromise by playing dress up when we get home.

I am a single mother of two beautiful little girls. I'm a college professor. Until I had my first child, I was a chaplain.

Three months into my first pregnancy, the constant and severe pain that ravaged my body changed everything. Every task—from walking, to sitting, to lifting the lightest of objects—left me in debilitating agony. Upon discovering that I had multiple and large fibroids, I was placed on bed rest and, with six months of bed rest ahead of me, then motherhood, it was time to surrender chaplaincy work for a while.

At my request, there was no gathering, or party, or community farewell at the end of my five-year stint. There was no cake, no card signed by two dozen staffers and no tearful goodbyes. I carried on my usual duties that day. Then I packed my items into two boxes, which a security guard deposited in the back seat of my car. I told everyone I'd be back as a volunteer as soon as I was able and I left. As it turned out, I would make many visits to The Space in the years to come, and still do to this day.

I convinced myself that I wasn't deeply saddened by this ending, that I should invest all of my energy in the new life brewing inside me. But this work was my calling and my heart's desire, and I was imagining my way back even as I left.

With a heavy heart and many unanswered questions, I was gone. I had a baby. Then another one. Then I left my partner, bought a condominium on the far side of town, and settled into teaching full-time and being a single mom.

One day I received a call on behalf of a resident at The Space. He had taken an art class, and was going to have a piece on display at an exhibit. He wanted me to come.

It was a crisp fall Sunday afternoon when my mother, my two daughters, and I loaded into the car and headed downtown to see the exhibit. As we entered the studio, I saw the resident who had invited me. The countless hours we'd spent together—and countless memories of prayers, conversations, hospital visits, and prayer services—filled my heart with an overwhelming sense of gratefulness and purpose, the same feeling I'd had on my first day of ministry.

Two years after that, I was invited to attend the annual memorial service at The Space to celebrate the lives of those who had died in the past year. It had been four years since I'd left The Space. I'd planned that memorial service every year while I was chaplain, and now I was watching the new chaplain—a joyful fifty-something-year-old vessel of God with salt-and-pepper hair and a starched white clerical collar over a black shirt. Her calm, soft voice and folded hands were a far cry from my wide-eyed over-exuberance.

Residents and staff members I had not seen for years warmly greeted me. After the service I jumped up to help serve food, and found that there were more than enough hands to do the job I most enjoyed—preparing and passing out heaping plates of food. So, instead, I settled into conversations with residents I remembered fondly.

It took only a few minutes before the conversations seemed to go back to just where they'd left off.

A resident who always wanted Reiki quickly found me and put in a request for an "appointment." I told her I was only visiting, but that didn't deter her. I told her I hadn't practiced for a long time, but that was of no consequence. I told her flatly I could not do it. She shook her head and continued pleading.

Another resident, who seemed annoyed with me for not being more assertive, wheeled his wheelchair away, looking back at me with an expression that was more akin to disgust than sympathy.

Yet another resident took my hand to say hello, then announced to everyone, including the new chaplain, that he had romantic dreams about me. I gently eased my hand away and smiled, feeling embarrassed, as if I had somehow nurtured this boundary breach.

Yet another resident became instantly annoyed with me when he informed me that he was dying, and I asked him if he was depressed. He looked me squarely in the eye and said, "I didn't say I was *depressed*, I said that I am dying! Those aren't the same thing, are they? Well, are they?"

"You're right," I said contritely. "They are not the same."

It was time for me to go. Not much had changed, except my ability to deal with these conversations constructively; that is, if I'd in fact ever had the ability at all.

It's a disorienting thing: to revisit a period in one's life, and to question if even a solitary remembrance is true.

When I started putting this project together in 2007, the AIDS pandemic had reached new heights, due, in part, to the residue of the Bush administration's policies that funded and promoted abstinence-first programs over condom distribution and needle exchange programs. According to Dr. Joseph Califano, founder of The National Center on Addiction and Substance Abuse at Columbia University, "Chemistry is chasing Christianity as the nation's largest religion," and millions of Americans, who daily take some kind of mood-altering, pain-killing, or mind-bending prescription drug, abuse alcohol and illegal drugs, and smoke cigarettes "likely exceed the number who weekly attend religious services." Califano also notes that drug abuse is now the leading perpetrator of new AIDS cases, with HIV infections as much as three times higher among methamphetamine users than among nonusers, and with intravenous drug users and their sexual partners spreading the disease. But Dr. Califano also notes that treatment and recovery is not as effective as it could be, in part because treatment communities attribute high dropout to individual addicts, with "problems within existing treatment systems contributing to the cycle of recovery and relapse." Furthermore, he notes, "Of those who enter therapeutic communities, 80 percent drop out within the first few months. Only 10 percent complete [lengthy] program[s]. Of that 10 percent, one-third are drug-free a year later, one-third are using at lower levels and a third are back to their pretreatment usage patterns."[1] Placing large pockets of socio-political responsibility for curbing the AIDS crisis on arbitrary pools of medically and psychologically compromised individuals liberates the rest of us from our moral and social obligation. It is, in fact, a retrospective and desperate position: *If you'd chosen not to*

1. Califano, *High Society*, 71

have sex, you would not have AIDS. If you'd chosen not to use drugs,
you would not have AIDS.

Among the lessons learned in my tenure as an HIV chaplain
is that stories can embody and express the angst of illness. Sharing
our reality is a form of agency.

In this vein I decided to extend the reach of these stories by
offering a course at the university titled "HIV/AIDS and Writing."
The purpose of the course was to encourage students to consider
the import of HIV/AIDS from within their current major areas
of study, and to consider how autopathography might be useful
across disciplinary interests. The class of twenty-three included
students majoring in biology, liberal studies, nursing, sociology,
English, and communications, among others. We started the class
reading about the history of the epidemic, then progressed to
memoirs and case studies written by caregivers, patients, doctors,
and mainstream press. By mid-semester, students started individual research on the virus that was relevant to their disciplinary
areas.

It was also at that mid-semester point when students made
their first visit to The Space, where they had the opportunity to
talk firsthand with residents. This was the place where theory and
practice met. There is nothing that prepares students to appreciate
the art of listening as acutely as academic practicums with human
subjects.

In "An Experiment in Teaching Empathy," Clinton Meek
concluded that if empathetic ability can be improved through
educational procedures—and his study seems to indicate that it
can—then "better measurements and demonstrations are needed
to indicate how we can teach empathy effectively."[2] These "better
measurements" were fully realized in the work of David Stockley,
who argued that having students learn entirely from texts gives
students no basis on which to identify with the experiences re-
corded in these texts; moreover, students have not been given the
pedagogical or philosophical information necessary to build iden-
tifications. Stockley defers to Tony Boddington—former director

2. Meek, "An Experiment in Teaching Empathy," 110.

of the British Schools Council—who believes that empathy, in the context of the school districts over which he has jurisdiction, is essential because it is "synonymous with identification, or the ability to enter into the minds and feelings of all the persons involved in an event."[3] In other words, such experiences round out the relationship between progressive pedagogies and radical empathy.

Even closer to the objective of my course was Douglas Bailey's essay titled "AIDS and American History: Four Perspectives on Experimental Learning," which offers an analysis of his efforts to create an interdisciplinary course that connects HIV/AIDS stories, collected locally, with the national landscape of HIV narratives. One of Bailey's guiding questions is "What can AIDS teach us about universal issues of sickness, healing, suffering, death and mourning? How can we communicate these experiences to the university and to the wider community?"[4] Through the course, he and his colleagues concluded that experiential learning allowed students to become a source of knowledge by learning history in their own community's context. Moreover, the course helped to establish "reciprocal relationships of knowledge and service between citizens outside the university and students and instructors associated with the university."[5] One course participant notes,

> I realized that historians still struggle to balance emotion with reason, sympathy with analysis, the heart with the head, in their teaching and writing. Achieving this balance is critical in understanding a controversial and emotionally compelling topic such as AIDS.[6]

Given the intersection of my beliefs both as professor and chaplain, I was provoked to ask, what paradigmatic interests are met through the use of HIV narratives? As a rhetorical event, the life stories of people with AIDS were as rich as the speeches of Abraham Lincoln or Frederick Douglass. As historical record, a

3. Stockley, "Empathetic Reconstruction in History and History Teaching," 53.

4. Bailey and DeVinny, "AIDS and American History," 1721.

5. Ibid., 1722.

6. Ibid., 1733.

narrative speaks as emphatically as any contemporary autobiography: after all, where is America's landscape more vividly depicted than through stories of suffering and triumph, marginality and spokesmanship?

Again, Douglas Bailey:

> Our class considered how to understand someone's story without reducing that person's experiences to a text to be analyzed. One especially perceptive student noted the distance he felt between [the subject's] experiences and his own experiences as someone who had never encountered AIDS first hand. He claimed that all that was possible was to listen to her story and try to sympathize with her problems. Other students disagreed and felt that the purpose of education was to develop the capacity to understand people with very different experiences and to analyze and interpret their words and actions.[7]

The long-term consequences of empathetic learning and practice extend far beyond my university's campus. The link between compassionate thinking and doing is—more and more—becoming the primary work of public historians, anthropologists, and sociologists. The possibilities for the use of narrative to promote engaged citizenry are boundless.

I hope that several decades from now I am standing side by side with my two adult daughters looking at an empty factory building that use to be The Space. I hope the need for this place and others like it will pass. When that happens, we will find other stories to tell, stories that—no doubt—will tether us to each other, and to our best selves, and to our world, in ways we cannot now imagine. In the words of Rumi, "Yesterday is gone and its tale is told. Today new seeds are growing."

Indeed, the seeds we plant, the seedlings we water, the vine we prune, the juice we press—these loved and cultivated buds—will become the wine we can drink.

I realize now that I was a servant in service to both the tellers and their stories. Through listening, I had the power to accept the

7. Ibid., 1730.

profane, the desperate, the triumphant, the shortcomings, and the celebrations, then to return them to the tellers respected, admired, appreciated, received.

Loved.

Normal.

Bibliography

Adams, Timothy Dow. *Telling Lies in Modern American Autobiography*. Chapel Hill, NC: University of North Carolina Press, 1990.

Andrews, Laurie. *HIV Care: A Comprehensive Handbook for Providers*. Thousand Oaks, CA: Sage, 1995.

Arbuckle, Gerald. *Healthcare Ministry: Refounding the Mission in Tumultuous Times*. Collegeville, MN: Liturgical, 2000.

Ariss, Robert M. *Against Death: The Practice of of Living with AIDS*. Sydney, Australia: Gordon and Breach, 1997.

Aronson, Jeffrey K. "Autopathography: the patient's tale." National Center for Biotechnology Information, National Institute of Health, v. 321 (7276) 1599–1602.

Atkinson, Paul, et. al. *Handbook of Ethnography*. London: Sage, 2001.

Bailey, Douglas, and Gabby DeVinny. "AIDS and American History: Four Perspectives on Experimental Learning." *The Journal of American History* 86 (2000) 1721–33.

Barks, Coleman, translator. *The Essential Rumi*. Edison: Castle, 1997.

Bartlett, John. *The Guide to Living with HIV Infection*. Baltimore: The Johns Hopkins University Press, 1991.

Bayer, Ronald. *AIDS Doctors: Voices from the Epidemic, An Oral History*. Oxford: Oxford University Press, 2000.

Bell McDonald, Katrina. *Embracing Sisterhood: Class, Identity, and Contemporary Black Women*, Lanham, Maryland: Rowman Littlefield, 2007.

Bond, George. *AIDS in Africa and the Caribbean*. Boulder, CO: Westview, 1997.

Califano, Joseph. *High Society: How Substance Abuse Ravages America and What to Do About It*. New York: Public Affairs, 2007.

Chris, Cynthia, ed. *Women, AIDS and Activism*. Boston: South End, 1990.

Cohen, Cathy. *The Boundaries of Blackness: AIDS and the Breakdown of Black Politics*. Chicago: University of Chicago Press, 1997.

Coles, Robert. *Children of Crisis: A Study of Courage and Fear*. Boston: Little Brown and Company, 1967.

———. *Doing Documentary Work*. Oxford: Oxford University Press, 1997.

———. *Women in Crisis: Lives of Struggle and Hope.* New York: Merloyd Lawrence, 1989.

Couser, G. Thomas. *Recovering Bodies: Illness, Disability and Life Writing.* Madison, WI: University of Wisconsin Press, 1997.

Daigle, Barbara. *HIV Homecare Handbook.* Sudbury, MA: Jones and Bartlett, 1999.

Dorn, Nicholas. *AIDS: Women, Drugs and Social Care.* London: Falmer, 1992.

Edgar, Timothy. *AIDS: A Communication Perspective.* Hillsdale, NY: Lawrence Erlbaum Associates, 1992.

Everist, Norma Cook, ed. *Ordinary Ministry, Extraordinary Challenges: Women and the Roles of Ministry.* Nashville: Abingdon, 2000.

Fee, Elizabeth. *AIDS: The Making of a Chronic Illness.* Berkeley, CA: University of California Press, 1992.

Fife, Wayne. *Doing Fieldwork: Ethnographic Methods for Research in Development Countries and Beyond.* New York: Palgrave MacMillan, 2005.

Frankl, Viktor. *Man's Search for Meaning.* New York: Simon and Schuster, 1984.

Giarelli, Jacobs LA. "Traditional healing and HIV-AIDS in KwaZulu-Natal, South Africa." *American Journal of Nursing 103* (2003) 36–46.

Gilbert, Dorie J. *African American Women and HIV/AIDS: Critical Responses.* Westport, Connecticut: Greenwood Group, 2003.

Goggin, Kathy, et al. "The Role of South African Traditional Health Practitioners in HIV/AIDS Prevention and Treatment." In *Globalization of HIV/ AIDS: An Interdisciplinary Reader,* edited by Robert Marlow, Cynthia Pope, and Renee White, 256–68. New York: Routledge, 2007.

Green, Edward. *AIDS and STDs in Africa: Bridging the Gap Between Traditional Healing and Modern Medicine.* Boulder, CO: Westview, 1994.

Groopman, Jerome, MD. *The Measure of Our Days.* New York: Viking, 1997.

Hanh, Thich Nhat. *Being Peace.* Berkeley, CA: Parallax, 1987.

Harper, Lynn. *Narrative, Health and Healing: Communication Theory, Research, and Practice.* Mahwah, NJ: Lawrence Erlbaum, 2005.

Henke, Suzette A. *Shattered Subjects: Trauma and Testimony in Women's Life-Writing.* New York: St. Martin's, 1998.

Herdt, Gilbert, and Shirley Lindenbaum. *The Time of AIDS: Social Analysis, Theory and Method.* London: Sage, 1992.

Herek, Gregory. *AIDS, Identity and Community.* Thousand Oaks, CA: Sage, 1995.

HIV/AIDS Surveillance Report, Center for Disease Control. Rev. ed. Atlanta: US Department of Health and Human Services (2007) 1–46.

Hoard, Ken. "To Have and Have Not." *A&U* 99 (January 2003) 42.

Jackson, W. Clay, MD. "Amlophagia Presenting as Gestational Diabetes." *Archives of Family Medicine,* 9 (2000) 649–52.

Kaplan, E. H., E. O'Keefe, and R. Heimer. "Evaluating the New Haven Needle Exchange Program." International Conference on AIDS, Yale School of Medicine 367 (June 16–18, 1991).

Kleinman, Arthur. *The Illness Narratives: Suffering, Healing and the Human Condition.* New York: Basic, 1988.

Kornfeld, Eve. "The Power of Empathy: A Feminist, Multicultural Approach to Historical Pedagogy." *The History Teacher* 26 (November 1992) 23–31.

Kubler-Ross, Elizabeth. *On Death and Dying.* New York: MacMillan, 1969.

Kuklin, Susan. *Fighting Back: What Some People Are Doing About AIDS.* New York: G. P. Putnam, 1989.

Lane, Sandra. "Needle Exchange: A Brief History." The Needle Exchange Program Evaluation Project. *The Kaiser Forums,* 1994.

Levine, Carol, ed. *Always on Call: When Illness Turns Families into Caregivers.* Nashville: Vanderbilt University Press, 2004.

Loseke, Donileen and James C. Cavendish. "Producing Institutional Selves: Rhetorically Constructing the Dignity of Sexually Marginalized Catholics." *Social Psychology Quarterly* 64, (December 2001) 347–62.

Mann, Cass. *The AIDS Cult: Essays on the Gay Health Crisis.* Provincetown, RI: Asklepios/Pagan, 1997.

Mars, Julie, ed. *A Little Book of Saints.* Kansas City, MO: Ariel, 1995.

Mattingly, Cheryl. *Narrative and the Cultural Construction of Illness and Healing.* Berkeley, CA: University of California Press, 2000.

McCollum, Audrey. *The Chronically Ill Child.* New Haven, CT: Yale University Press, 1981.

Meek, Clinton R. "An Experiment in Teaching Empathy." *Journal of Educational Sociology* 31 (1957) 107–10.

Milner, Callie. "Childhood, Interrupted." *A&U* 9 (2003) 38–39 Publishers, 2008.

Mintz, Susannah B. *Unruly Bodies: Life Writing by Women with Disabilities.* Chapel Hill, NC: University of North Carolina Press, 2007

Moffitt, Catherine. "The Relationship Between Burnout and Self-Esteem in Nurses." Thesis, the School of Graduate Studies in Behavioral Science, Southern Connecticut State University, 1996.

Monette, Paul. *Borrowed Time: An AIDS Memoir.* New York: Harcourt Brace Jovanovich, 1988.

New York State Department of Health AIDS Institute. "HIV and Smoking: A Wake Up Call for Action." *Light Up Your Life, A Leadership Forum on HIV and Smoking* (2006) 1–8.

O'Brien, Mary Elizabeth. *A Sacred Covenant: The Spiritual Ministry of Nursing.* Sudbury: Jones and Bartlett.

Oppenheimer, Joshua. *Acting on AIDS: Sex, Drugs and Politics.* London: Serpent's Tail, 1997.

Perloff, Richard. *Persuading People to Have Safer Sex: Applications of Social Science to the AIDS Crisis.* Mahwah, NJ: Lawrence Erlbaum Associates, 2001.

Pila of Hawaii. *The Secrets and Mysteries of Hawaii.* Deerfield Beach, FL: Health Communications, Inc., 1995.

Reynolds, Dale. "Contextual Clues." *A&U* Issue 99 (January 2003) 33–35.

Resnik, Susan. *Blood Saga: Hemophilia, AIDS and the Survival of a Community.* Berkeley, CA: University of California Press, 1999.

Saunders, Cicely. *Living with Dying.* Kent: Oxford Medical, 1989.

Schernhammer, Eva S. and Graham A. Colditz. "Suicide Rates Among Physicians: A Qualitative and Gender Assessment (Meta-Analysis)." (December 2004), 2295–2302. (Viewed online at http://ajp.psychiatryonline.org/cgi/content/full/ajp;161/12/2295).

Selwyn, Peter A. *Surviving the Fall: The Personal Journey of an AIDS Doctor.* New Haven, CT: Yale University Press, 1998.

Shepard, Benjamin Heim. *White Nights and Ascending Shadows: An Oral History of the San Francisco AIDS Epidemic.* London: Cassell, 1997.

Sipe, Rebecca Bowers. "Academic Service Learning: More than Just Doing Time." The English Journal 90, no. 5, The School and the Community. (May 2001) 33–38.

Stockley, David. "Empathetic Reconstruction in History and History Teaching." *History and Theory,* Vol. 22, No. 4 Beiheft 22: The Philosophy of History Teaching (December 1983) 50–65.

Stringer, Ernie, et al. *Community Based Ethnography: Breaking Traditional Boundaries of Research, Teaching and Learning.* Mahwah, NJ: Lawrence Erlbaum Associates, 1997.

"What Can We Expect from Substance Abuse Treatment?" (Part of IDV/HIV Prevention Series) Center for Disease Control, Department of Health and Human Services, February 2002 (http:www.cdc.gov/idv/facts/expectationsfin.pdf), 2.

www.ingramcontent.com/pod-product-compliance
Lightning Source LLC
Chambersburg PA
CBHW032354280326
41935CB00008B/565